DINNER W̶ ... RS
A TRUE STOR... ...RY

BY C... ...ELLS

Dear Richard,

Thinking of you and
wishing you wellness.

Kindly,
Colleen Wells

May 29, 2015
Louisville, KY

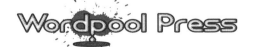

Colleen Wells believes the health of the planet impacts humanity's collective mental health.

That is why a portion of the proceeds of this book will be donated to Earth Charter Indiana.

The mission of the Earth Charter Initiative is to actively participate, in a systemic and integrated way, in the present transition to sustainable ways of living on the planet, founded on a shared ethical framework that includes respect and care for the community of life, ecological integrity, universal human rights, respect for diversity, social and economic justice, democracy, and a culture of peace.

www.earthcharterindiana.org

Wordpool Press
10970 196th Ave.
Big Rapids, MI 49307

www.wordpoolpress.com
wordpoolsubmissions@gmail.com

Published by: Wordpool Press
Original Cover Art by: Kristin Llamas
Wells, Colleen, Dinner with Doppelgangers: A True Story of
Madness and Recovery

ISBN-10: 0990588823
ISBN-13: 978-0-9905888-2-5

10 9 8 7 6 5 4 3 2 1
1. mental illness 2. memoir

First Edition
Ordering Information:
Quantity sales. Special discounts are available on quantity
purchases by corporations, associations, and others. For details,
contact the publisher at the address above.

Printed in the United States of America

If you desire healing,
let yourself fall ill
let yourself fall ill.
— Rumi

For Rick, my love and my rock, and Yakob and Ayalkbet, who taught my heart to sing. And for Gaelle who, while not a part of *this* story, is my daughter who deserves a book all her own.

ACKNOWLEDGEMENTS

Make no bones about it: I know who my cheerleaders are. I am blessed with wonderful family and friends, but for this memoir a heartfelt thanks goes out to my brother, Todd Fearrin, who is always there for me in a pinch; Uncle Terry Boden; Aunts Patty Sampson and Jane York; friends Susan Edwards, Kristin Llamas, and Michele McColligan; and especially my husband, Rick Wells, and our sons, Yakob and Ayalkbet. Many of you helped during acute manic episodes of my illness or when the weight of depression was too heavy to bear.

I'd like to express my sincere gratitude to all of my parents: Carol and Bob Fearrin, who did their best to care for me both in 1988, when being diagnosed with bipolar disorder (then termed manic depression, which wasn't common in adolescents), and later as an adult, and Jan and John Caton for always encouraging my writing and for rooting for me even when it was hard.

I shared some of my earlier work about this subject with professors at Indiana University and Butler University. For those experiences I am grateful. I'd also like to extend gratitude to the Spalding University MFA program faculty and staff, especially mentors Dianne Aprile, Robert Finch, and Richard Goodman. I appreciate my many readers at various stages of the book, with a special thanks to Christine Brandel, Betty Hawes, and Carol Werner. I am grateful for the support of my writers' group comprised of Molly Gleeson, Jonathan Holland, and Cara Prill. Molly Peacock and long-time mentor Jim Poyser gave me the encouragement to make this idea for a book take flight. Without Ellie Bryant's razor-sharp eye and gentle wisdom, it wouldn't exist.

Portions of this book have been published in *Deltona Howl*, *The Voices Project*, *Vine Leaves Literary Journal*, *The Barefoot Review*, *Psychic Meatloaf*, *Adoptive Families Magazine*, *Muscadine Lines*, *The Petigru Review*, *New Southerner*, *VerbSap*, *Georgetown Review*, *NUVO*, *Chicken Soup for the Adopted Soul*, *In Other Words: An American Poetry Anthology*, *jmww*, *Firestories: Further Thoughts on Radically Rethinking Mental Illness*, *(T)HERE: Writings on Returnings*, *Potomac Review*, and *Veils, Halos and Shackles: International Poetry on the Abuse and Oppression of Women*.

A NOTE TO THE READER

I have struggled for many years to give voice
and form to my experience with bipolar disorder
I, which is different from bipolar II and other
mood disorders. While doing some research
at the bookstore in the young adult section, I
stumbled upon a book called *I Don't Want to Be
Crazy* by Samantha Schutz. The young woman
had penned a memoir-in-verse about her battle
with anxiety. In all my years of schooling, I
had never even known such a species of book
existed.

While this is not a collection of poetry, sharing
my experience in small pieces seemed like an
appropriate way to attempt to tell my story. This
true story begins with a young adult's voice,
progresses as I grow up, and changes colors
with the roller coaster of my disorder.

Although this book is largely chronological,
bipolar disorder is messy, especially during
periods of time when I was hospitalized and my
mind veered in too many directions to record
all of them here. Patients came and went from
the hospitals, some repeatedly, like me. My
experiences do not necessarily reflect those of
all people with a bipolar I diagnosis. Symptoms
vary widely from individual to individual.

In service to the reader, I have created the best path toward understanding, with snapshots of my life with this disease. I have changed names and/or identifying characteristics in instances where I thought it necessary. Memoir is a tricky beast. How do you separate fact from fiction when everyone views life through a unique lens? I have had conversations with writers who have different viewpoints, and the consensus has been to tell the truth in the best damn way you can, find freedom in it, and worry about what to call it later. Philosophies aside, this much I know to be true: it takes a lot of courage to tell your true story.

While bipolar I and II affect roughly two percent of the population, it touches the lives of many more people, including family, friends, and healthcare workers. My goal in writing this book is to share my story (and subsequently my hope) with everyone impacted by this disease.

-ONE-

High School

My high school days are like a country song.
Whiskey and beer, cheating and heartache.

Even then, although I didn't know it,
I was slipping.

Eighteen

I am eighteen.
The summer following graduation, I grow
forgetful and anxious. My friends can't wait to
go off to college, but I don't even know how to
do my own laundry.

As summer progresses, I won't get out of my
pink canopy bed. My friends are worried. My
hair splays across the pillow, a greasy mess.

1

My pink phone goes unanswered. The ring
sounds muffled, as if submerged in water.

I can't eat. I can't sleep. I won't bathe.
I am wasted—
wasting away.

Stranger's Got a Gun

My family doctor prescribes amitriptyline, but
I'm still not right. A reoccurring thought tells me
traveling to Florida will make it better. I spend
my graduation money on a plane ticket.

There I do some things uncharacteristic of me,
like walking onto a dock and inviting myself to
go deep-sea fishing with a group of strangers.
I reel in a huge kingfish but have to throw it
back due to regulations.

After the fishing expedition, one of the strangers
gives me a ride back to my condo. I talk
him into buying me a six-pack because I am
underage.

While he's inside the gas station, I open his
glove box, find a gun. It's black and not that
small. I want to pick it up, but instinct stops me.

When the stranger drops me off, he orders me to

go right inside and be careful with the beer.
He knows something about me is off.
There's something not right about him too.
I feel like telling him to be careful with the gun,
but instinct stops me.

Poison

I notice food at home takes on a strange,
metallic taste.

Crystal Light tastes even more chemical
than usual.

It occurs to me I am being poisoned.

My Doctor

That first night in the hospital I meet my doctor.
He wears a tie with dolphins on it and top siders.
I decide this is a good sign, but then he tells me
I am a very sick girl.

So how can he make me better?
And how long will it take?

Group

In the morning they give me more Haldol,
which winds me up like a spinning top, like a

whirling dervish in a blue, terrycloth bathrobe.

After breakfast it is time for group. Our plastic
chairs in primary colors are fashioned into a half
circle. I am told to sit down. All eyes are on me.
Everyone is dressed for the day but me. I turn to
the woman to my right and ask her if we are in
hell and if she sees the black ravens hovering in
the sky like I do. She gets up, takes another seat.

I am left alone, in group.

Borderline Personality Disorder

That summer and fall I am in and out of the
hospital a lot. I collect diagnoses
like I used to collect flavored lip gloss.
Depression.
Major depression.
Manic depression.

My favorite is borderline personality disorder.
I am borderline. My personality is disorderly.

Seeing Red

My mental maladies are taxing my mother.

We're on our way to outpatient therapy.
Mom is driving fast. When a signal turns red,

she yells at me that I made her miss the light. Her face and the stop light are the same color. I'm not sure if she's mad at me, or mad at herself.

Little Green Man

My friend, Brad, thinks getting out will help and takes me to Indianapolis. Downtown, we happen upon a homeless man. His toilet paper is poking out of the army-green knapsack he's wearing across his back. There's something wild in his eyes, and he sees something in mine too.

He says, "Sister, there's a little green man in my head too. If you don't like yours, tell him to fuckin' get out." Then he runs off.

I tell Brad I want to follow and begin to hurry after him, but Brad pulls me back. I watch as the man disappears from my line of sight, hungering for more of his wisdom.

Ode to Marla

Marla and I have in common sun-kissed, bleached hair, a peer group, and smoking menthol cigarettes. Her punk eighties haircut and amazingly large earrings are hallmarks of her style which garners her attention when she moves to our small, conservative town.

Some of it she doesn't mind,
some of it she does.

Now she's heading to Rhode Island for school.

One of my closest friends is moving the farthest
away. But it's not just that. Marla's a nurturer
and a rock. This loss…it hurts.

My Favorite Blue Jeans

I am placed on the adolescent ward where Alice
won't eat, and Rose had a miscarriage, and
Steve overturns chairs until he gets a shot in the
ass.

My favorite blue jeans go missing. I know it
was Rose. Dark eyes always staring, hair shaved
on top with a long tail in back giving her the
appearance of a newt.

I go into her room and get them back, but I am
the one in trouble. They put me on "level one"
where I must sit on a hard chair and face the
wall and think about why I'm here.

Later I'll have to atone for my behavior
in a group of peers.

The longer I'm on the chair,
the less I know what I'll say.

Queen

In the hospital they use the words "processing feelings" a lot. Makes me think of processing meat.

I tell them my story. My parents divorce when I am out of diapers but not out of the stage where they are my whole world. Not long afterward my mom remarries a widower with four children.

There are a lot of rules in this new family, like we have to say, "Yes, Ma'am," and "Yes, Sir," which wouldn't feel so weird if we lived in the South. The rules for my stepsiblings aren't always the same as mine. I think that's why they call me "Colleen the Queen." For example, when it's time to clean my stepdad's office I'm asked to do simple tasks like straighten the magazines and wash the coffee mugs while my stepsiblings get the hard jobs like vacuuming and dusting. And I know they're hard because there are a lot of desks to dust, and I can hear their huffs as they plunk the sweeper down the stairs.

But I don't make up the rules,
and it isn't my fault.
I do make up a song, though,
with only two lines:
I'm lonely, I'm lonely,
Nobody likes me.

And I'd gladly give up my crown
if it meant they'd like me.

Baby Sisters in the Bassinet

Mom was pregnant, and when the twins, Sarah
Jane and Emily Elizabeth, died, my brother
tells me she laid them in a white bassinet for
viewing.

I don't remember. But I can still hear her
screaming in the night while we kids hid in our
beds. I remember my stepdad calling a friend
for help.

And her going away.
And coming home.
But not the same.

I was sad for Mom, but sad for me too. I wanted
to know if this meant we wouldn't get to watch
Sonny and Cher anymore while she brushed my
hair.

Sunday School

We always go to church on Sunday, which is boring but okay because we get doughnuts and juice afterwards in the parish basement.

Sometimes, after church, my stepdad reads to us from the Bible, then asks questions. I don't always understand what he reads, but I try to think of answers, because I'm wedged on the big, faux leather couch between two siblings, and the more questions that are asked, the longer we get to hang out together.

Do the Math

Not long after the twins die, Mom gets pregnant again. She has two girls over the next two years.

My dad remarries. They have two kids—a girl and a boy. I now have four steps and four halves, but no full-blooded siblings.

I would have been happy with just one—'cuz blood is thicker than water, and two is a better number than eight.

I don't see my dad as often as I'd like to growing up. Sometimes I wonder how different things might be if I lived with him. I think about

that a lot, but realistically the math would've
come up the same.

TV

I have a little black and white TV in my room.
Some movies leave scars deeply embedded in
my psyche, like the film *Roots* because of the
meanness of the masters and the way they break
up families.

Another is a show about a woman who's a little
slow but dreams of being a mom. They want to
sterilize her against her will, and I had to turn it
off after that.

It makes me wonder if one day when I'm older
I could lose my mind and more...

Hello, Joe

We have a myna bird named Joe in the corner
of our dining room. His shiny, black feathers
are littered with dandruff, the floor and bars of
his cage are splattered in poop.

He repeats what he hears, things like, "Hello,
Joe" and "What the hell are you doing?"

We shouldn't have a dirty bird where we eat.

And anyway, my name is not Joe.
And I have no idea what I'm doing.

I Want My MTV

Susan's mom and my mom were friends back in
the day and were even pregnant with us at the
same time, which makes Susan and me sort of
like sisters.

Mary Ellen and Mom went their separate ways,
as grownups sometimes do, then were surprised
when they ended up living across the street from
each other years later.

As Susan and I forge our own friendship, we
become inseparable. Being her friend comes
with benefits: we can have Buddig meats
covered with Cheez Whiz to make sandwiches,
and she's also got cable TV.

We love the VJ Martha the most because she's a
wannabe rocker like us. Martha shows us Pat
Benatar, Lita Ford, Madonna, and The Go-Go's,
which we like because we want to be strong
women like them.

Every day after school, I want to eat Buddig
with my bud, and I want my MTV too.

Dinner Is Served

Sometimes for meals Mom makes us fish sticks
and tater tots. Then she and my stepdad
sit down to steak and baked potatoes.
I don't really know what I'm missing,
yet something here is missing.

Small Zoo

I have a small zoo in my room—an ant farm,
gerbils, goldfish, and Sea-Monkeys. After my
gerbils (who are thought to both be males) have
babies, I awake one morning to discover that the
heads of the tiny creatures had been chewed off,
probably by the mother.

I scream for my parents. My stepdad takes care
of the carnage.

When I come home from school, the whole cage
is gone, along with any evidence of the demise
of half a dozen gerbil children.

Merry Prankster

I like to play pranks on Susan. Sometimes they
are simple, like hiding an egg in the back of
her dresser drawer, waiting for her to complain
about the smell.

And sometimes they're more elaborate,
like when I stuffed some of my stepdad's
clothes with newspaper, affixing a cut-out of
John Stamos' face on top with tape, and sat my
scarecrow in an armchair. The final touch was
placing a notebook in his lap, where I wrote a
sexual comment about my fake John Stamos.

Then I hauled it across the street, placed it on
Susan's doorstep, rang the doorbell, and hid.

Unfortunately, Susan didn't answer the door.
Her older sister did, who yelled, "What the
hell?!"

This attracted Susan's dad. Let's just say he was
not pleased. Later, when he found out it was me,
he threatened to tell my mom.

Luckily, he didn't, but I was left to wonder
about my actions. My punishment was in
knowing normal teens don't usually go to these
extremes to pull a prank.

Summertime and the Livin' Is Almost Easy

In the summers, we go to the lake cottage for
long periods of time. We can have one paper
grocery sack for packing our clothes, and I'm
not allowed to talk too much during the drive

because my stepdad doesn't like it, especially when I pretend my fingers are people and start chatting with them.

I sit by the water and read under big, old trees whose roots are never thirsty 'cuz they're close enough to the lake for a sip. My friends are the characters in my books: Runaway Ralph, Ramona and Beezus, Amelia Bedelia, Charlie Bucket, and Nancy Drew, changing with my age.

At night, when our parents take the boat to visit friends who live across the lake, we sneak bread slathered with sugar and cinnamon. My brother climbs the rafters like a stealthy cat, and the older kids tell me ghost stories outside in the dark.

Someone is always on the lookout for the glowing lights of the boat, and for a while I feel like I'm part of something. But then we see the tell-tale orange and scatter to our bunk beds because we know we'll get in trouble for still being up. My heart thumps as I get into fake sleep mode. My heart hopes our parents will go out again soon.

Anger Management

But telling my story isn't enough. I must act it out, get in touch with my anger.

In the hospital, we have a special room with a blue wrestling mat and some mallets that look like Popeye's arms. I have to swing them against the mat and yell at the same time.

When I process my anger, it makes my doctor happy. I know he might lift a restriction for my work or maybe even move me to another level.

But I don't feel angry,
I feel empty.

Who Am I?

In here, not only do I miss my family and friends, I miss myself.

But who am I?

Molly Ringwald and the Brat Pack, MTV and wanting to be Madonna, Michael Jackson, Prince, Bon Jovi. I am a teenager in the eighties, a child of privilege growing up amidst cornfields and railroad tracks in a ritzy neighborhood on the reservoir. Long, cable-knit sweaters, bobbed hair, big hair, Swatch watches in every color.

Guns N' Roses and tight Guess jeans, metal band concerts and braces, sneaking cigarettes in the side yard while contemplating the moon. Riding with the windows down, air against my cheek, the thump of AC/DC humming up around us.

Cutting up in choir, exchanging notes in class, the electricity in the parking lot when school lets out. Jim Beam whiskey burning the back of my throat, skipping curfew to play euchre, Budweisers and the right bower.

Meeting a boy on the golf course, heart thumping from the thrill of getting away unseen, heart thumping from his touch. Recounting what happened on the fifth hole to Susan. The trilling pink telephone by my bed, hoping it's the boy from the golf course, talking all night.

Waterskiing at dawn, the lake smooth as a skipping stone. Sitting on Marla's roof, the stars so close they look like I can grab them.

In here, I can't see any stars, just the fluorescent ceiling lights. It's like my own light has gone out.

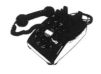

-TWO-

Staff Talks

On the adolescent ward, you get two staff talks
a day. One evening, I'm talking to a technician
named Keith who looks up or side to side but
never directly at me. He's got big grey-blue eyes
behind silver glasses, runs his fingers through
his curly hair a lot. It's like he's with me but not
really present.

One night, he asks me if I try to get my way in
life by using my body. I don't know if this is
sexual harassment, but it doesn't feel right to
me. His eyes lock with mine and I shake my
head, "no."

Inside, I'm shaking too.

Fear

Sometimes I get scared. Circling around the nurses' station I ask if I'll ever get better. It doesn't help that I've heard them whispering about long-term care in conjunction with my name.

I know these places. Central State is haunted with former residents who probably died of suicide or abuse. Or maybe broken hearts. Then there's Larue Carter, which is probably scary too. But they tell me not to worry. That it's like the popular song by Bobby McFerrin, "Don't Worry, Be Happy." Only I can't stop worrying, and I can't be happy.

I don't know what long term means for sure, but I think it means I might be there forever, because some people are broken and can't be fixed.

It's Weird to Me...

It's weird to think that on other floors women are having babies, people are dying, and there's all sorts of emergencies.

While I'm tucked away on a locked ward where I'm not pregnant or dying.

I'm not even on suicide precautions.
I just am.

Level Three

Somehow, though, I've made it to level three.
I can go in the music room and listen to my
approved cassette tapes. I'm disappointed when
my Grateful Dead tape isn't approved, but Ted,
another patient, has Guns N' Roses. We listen to
"Sweet Child O' Mine" over and over.

In the song, the singer sings of not ever wanting
to witness the tiniest bit of sadness in his former
lover's blue eyes.

I wonder who's looking out for the pound of
pain in mine.

Room Confinement

My doctor lets me out on pass to see how I
function in the real world. Upon my return I
smuggle cigarettes onto the ward, lighting up in
the music room.

Ted uses the space after me, rats me out to the
nurses.

I am placed in confinement in a bare room near

the nurses' station. There's nothing to do in here except peel the plastic baseboards. When this gets old, I start singing "Nuttin' for Christmas."

I might not be getting anything for Christmas, but you can bet I'll be getting additional meds real soon.

Recreational Therapy

Sometimes in RT we play the spoon game where we chant: "This is how we play the spoon game, the spoon game, the spoon game…" while passing the spoon around the circle. When the leader stops the chant, whoever has the spoon has to do something with it. Then we all follow suit for another round.

When Doug gets the spoon, he places it on his nose for a good long while.

But my nose is pug and when it's my turn it doesn't stay on very long.

I'm worried about when I have to go, 'cuz I want to do something clever, so these people will like me.

Phone Calls

Steve, the guy who gets shots in the ass
sometimes, likes my mom. He has something
like a speech impediment. When he means to
say "Dang!" it comes out as "Dag!"

For example, when Mom drops off some
laundry, he says to her, "Dag, nice dress!"

Steve has no one to reach out to when it's time
for phone calls, so I give him our home number.

Now Mom is getting calls from two mental
patients.

Major Depression

When my doctor comes I get nervous. First
he chats up the nurses, then skims my chart,
running his pointer finger down the page as he
reads. I try to think of good things to say for our
talk. Things about feelings. But I'm distracted
when I see the label on the side of my chart says
"Major Depression" where it used to say just
"Depression."

He thinks I'm getting worse. What's the next
level of depression after "Major"? Will I be First
Lieutenant Colonel of Depression?

Postcards from the Edge

I love when the mail comes. Today there is a letter from my little sister, Robin. She says that she misses me, and even loves me, but she is enjoying wearing my clothes. It is one of the sweetest things I've ever read, and I don't even mind about the clothes. Because I bet that means she's forgiven me for the time I called the police on myself when the depression wouldn't stop. If it wouldn't go away, I would.

The patrol car screeched to a halt in front of our house, just as my little sister and her friends were boarding the bus.

I must have scared her. I must have shamed her. Little gawkers, big sister's off her rocker.

The Creep

Back home, sadness creeps in. It cannot be lured away by swimming in our pool or listening to Prince while gazing up at the top of my canopy bed where I used to hang pictures of him.

Instead, I stay indoors, pacing like an expectant father. Only I've got no reason to pace, and when I try to get my legs to stop, they don't listen.

Three

My parents are eating their dinner when I walk into the dining room and stare. I want them to know I am still sick. That I don't understand what has happened to me. Mostly, I just want them to fix it.

I begin to do laps around the table. My stepdad sets down his fork and looks at me in frustration. He asks me how old I am to act this way.

"Three," I say. "I am three."

The Bubble

My face feels tight like I'm wearing a dried mask. It's the Mellaril. My thoughts feel heavy too. I decide to end them like I've seen done on TV.

I sit in my 1971 Pacer with the Native American design on the seats. My friends call it the Bubble. The garage door is closed, but I've left my window open a little while I think some more about if I really want to do this. Not long after I turn on the car, my Aunt Patty, who is visiting, finds me listening to Elton John in my Bubble.

She is upset. I have made a mess again. When my mom gets home, they decide I need to go back.

-THREE-

PICU (Psychiatric Intensive Care Unit)

My mom is on one side, a cop on the other.
The cop asks me why a pretty girl like me wants
to kill herself. I can't make words. I am dirty
and shedding like an animal. Dislodged hairs
have fallen all over my red Forenza sweater.

He drops me off at PICU. Sarah greets me
by throwing a flower pot at my head. She is
restrained. Two orderlies carry her to a room
where she gets a shot.

They notice me watching in the doorway and
tell me if I don't get out that I'll be next.

In the dayroom there is Ginny. She shuffles
when she walks. Ginny keeps saying, "Roy
Rogers and Dale Evans are coming to town" and
that "we're having Big Mac soup for lunch."

An elderly man dozes in a chair. When he wakes up he is laughing.

Green Jell-O

Breakfast is not as good in PICU as it is on the other wards. It's like they're giving us whatever they can find.

Today's meal includes green Jell-O, milk, and a hard-boiled egg. I stare at the smiling missing child on my milk carton, wonder where she is, wonder where I am.

Two Minds

I hear from one of the nurses that some of my friends have caused a ruckus when they tried to see me and weren't let in. This makes me sad because I miss them and happy because they tried. Happy or sad. Sad or happy. Which is it?

The Smokes Are on Me

At least in PICU you can smoke.
But the carton my mom brings gets stolen.
It was locked up in the special cabinet
that we have to ask staff to unlock.

Smoke 'em if you got 'em,

and I don't got 'em anymore.

Waiting for My Doctor

My doctor in PICU speaks broken English.
His hair is covered in a white turban.
It looks like the top of an ice cream cone.

At the end of one conversation, I am baffled
when he says he's ordering me a pregnancy test.
But most days he doesn't show up at all.

Posey

Somehow Steve winds up in PICU too. We
play tricks on the staff. One morning when the
attendant asks me if I know my name and what
day it is, I pretend not to hear him.

But the joke is on me because he gets frustrated
and says, "Maybe this will help you remember,"
then places me in the Posey. The Posey looks
like an airplane seat only it has restraints for
your wrists to be bound to the arms of the chair.
"Dag!" Steve yells. "She didn't do nuthin'!" As
I sit there for hours, I wish I had answered his
questions.

Lithium

I am back upstairs on the adolescent ward, lying
in bed with my arms out to my side. Nearby a
woman holds a plastic tub filled with needles
and vials. Another one finds the vein she has
been looking for, pats it with her finger, cleanses
the spot, and sticks the needle in.
They are preparing me for lithium.

For several months I've been in and out of
the hospital, and I get the diagnosis of manic
depression in near lock-stop timing of when the
insurance money runs out.

Cold Air

The cold air hits me. I have spent the warmest
months indoors, but I am free to go home. My
friends have finished their first semester at
school. I see them and realize how they have
gone on without me. But they are still my
friends.

They don't judge me, and when we get together,
it's like no time has passed at all.
Maybe, just maybe, I'm cured.

Celebrities

At home, we don't talk about the hospital, but my mom gives me books. One is a big, brown technical text called *Manic Depression*. Another is a memoir by Patty Duke Astin, who is manic-depressive like me.

I discover there are other celebrities who are reported to have unstable moods, like Margot Kidder and Carrie Fisher. But they are celebrities, and I am not famous. Being in their company doesn't make me feel any better.

Janie

I attend a manic-depressive support group. The leader, Janie, who is also manic-depressive, takes me under her wing.

She's a mental health advocate. It's her job to make sure places like Central State Hospital have enough chairs.

I know some day, some way, I want to be an advocate too. And I want to do more than count chairs.

Feedback

I get so excited about my hospital writings that
I call my old high school English teacher, Miss
Flatt.

In school, I could tell she was one of the
teachers who cared about her students.

She reads what I have written with enthusiasm,
which makes me happy because I am always
starving for feedback.

Food for Thought

It doesn't help my weight that I'm working
at two fast food restaurants. Chili dogs and
cheeseburgers, sundaes and spaghetti over ten
minute breaks.

This is not the life I planned for myself.

I should be done with a year of school,
but it seems instead, I've enrolled
in the school of hard knocks.

-FOUR-

Sister Lith

In August, I join my friends at college in Bloomington. I try to keep up with them. Try to take a full load, but I drop two classes.

I trust my new doctor at the health center, tell him I don't like taking my lithium, that it means I'm different. He tells me he takes insulin for his diabetes, and he doesn't like it either. I keep taking my medicine, joking to Susan that my name is "Sister Lith."

Serenade

My ex from high school
lives one story above me in the dorm.

He plays Led Zeppelin on his guitar.
I wish it was for me.

Mail

I check the mail hoping for money from my
mom or my dad. Instead, there's a form letter
stating Janie has taken her life. It turns out she,
who had assisted so many, couldn't help herself.

Somewhere I've read about the rate of suicide
in manic-depressives, but statistics are just
numbers. I've been to Janie's house, even toured
Central State with her once.
This is real.

And it sucks.

Denver

One summer, when I'm no longer living in the
dorms, I pick up a free Australian shepherd.
She's black with charcoal baby eyes, and I name
her Denver after a character in a book I read for
school. I take her home to show Mom.

My puppy zips in circles through the yard.
Later, Mom is bringing in my small nieces
from boating on the lake, hollering for me to
help them dock.

I leave Denver in the yard, thinking I should tie
her leash to something, but Mom says to hurry.

When I finish my task of helping the little ones off the boat, I can't find Denver.

Then I see her leash stuck between two boards of the pier. When I pull up the leash my puppy hangs from it, contorted like a wet towel extracted from the washer.

Mom rocks the dead dog as I run off screaming. Later she tries to appease me with a squirming black Lab whom I know I'll never love and who gets returned to the breeder.

Comfortably Numb

All I can think to do is escape, pack my ruby-colored VW bus, this time heading East, to Marla's house.

On the way out of town, I pick up an unwanted coonhound, call her Annie. The dog is skittish, and I can tell she's been through some stuff. She rides shotgun, ears flapping in the wind, as we zoom through the mountains listening to "Peace Frog" cranked up on the Pioneer.

The beat of the song, the rhythm of the road, and Shotgun Annie at my side effectively numb my pain.

Bus Driver

One of my jobs in college is to drive for DSS,
Disabled Student Services.

I drive for the wheelchair bound chancellor,
Herman B. Wells, and an artist who is also a
paraplegic, and a blind professor who makes
me count the steps from his door to where I've
parked.

One. Two. Three. Four. Five. Six.
This job makes me realize I could have it worse.

Deal

I'm on academic probation because I'm weak
in math and science. I switch my major a few
times, elementary education, psychology, even
English, but I still must pass basic biology.

I struggle to learn Mendel's peas and get a tutor,
which doesn't help. Finally, I approach my
professor who asks what I'm good at. When I
tell him I like writing, he says he'll make me a
deal that I write papers instead of take exams,
which helps me pass his course, which helps me
stay in school.

Maybe my ability to problem solve and be

resourceful means I'm not still sick.
Maybe I am well.

Freedom

Annie's favorite thing, besides riding shotgun, is
running wild through the woods at Lake Griffy.
The second I unclamp her leash, she takes off
with the speed of a greyhound.

I follow her into the woods, hear her feet
thumping down the path as she disappears.
In moments like this, we are both free.

The Break-in

Susan's roommate, Adrienne, wants to quit her
lease, but their landlord won't let her. So she
stages a break-in, writes stuff with lipstick on
her mirror.

I'm at home in Noblesville, visiting my family
and doing laundry, when a cop calls, asks if it
was me. Apparently she told them it could have
been me because I'm manic-depressive.

I didn't know Adrienne very well, but I do now.

Five Minutes to Worry

Once, when I was telling my therapist about my worries, she fell asleep.

In another session, the best advice she gave me was to pick a time each day for five minutes to worry, and not to do it until then.

Shotgun Annie Has a Friend

I work at an Italian restaurant called Grisanti's where I meet Michele. She's quirky and has had her own ups and downs. We become fast friends.

She gets a German shepherd named Althea. Now Shotgun Annie has a friend.

Burning Down the House

I decide on a whim to tell a guy I'd been seeing that I have manic depression. He asks me if that means I am going to burn down his house.

I don't see him after that. And another new friend that I met in summer classes, who introduced us, doesn't call me anymore.

The Scythe

During college, I see lots of Dead shows with friends. Me and Julie, one of my best friends from high school and now college, are camping after a concert and realize the van is out of gas. Nobody else will wake up, so we walk out of the campgrounds in search of petrol. We get terribly lost in a rural area in Ohio. A truck passes us slowly, turns around, comes back.

We get in, and he promises he'll take us to get gas. But we keep driving farther out, with no civilization in sight.

He says he's just got to go to his barn
to get a scythe for his brother.
We scream for him to let us out.
When he slows down, I open the passenger
door. We tumble out and run. Eventually, we
find a gas station and our way back.

I always wonder what would have happened
at the man's barn.

I've made lots of bad decisions, but jumping
from his truck was one of the good ones.

Grunge Babies

Michele and I are each dating younger guys.
They're musicians with lots of tattoos and
piercings that make them look like bad boys, but
mine has a soft voice and eyes that truly smile.

He calls me his "fucking babe" and means it in a
good way.

We love them more than we should,
and we call them the Grunge Babies.

Depakote

I take lithium for nearly a decade. It has allowed
me to graduate and take jobs. But it doesn't help
with the depression I sometimes get. I switch to
Depakote, a salmon-colored pill.

The side effects of Depakote can be
somnolence, nausea, diarrhea, dizziness, weight
gain, and hair loss, not to mention liver failure.

As with lithium, my doctor orders blood draws,
which I hate, but the functioning of my liver is
just as important as the functioning of my brain.

-FIVE-

The Depakote Years

The Depakote years are good ones. I land a
great job in Indianapolis, start graduate school,
and find my soulmate, Rick, sitting at his desk.

He is my boss. He writes poetry
and shows it to nobody but me.

This Love

Rick leaves me messages all around like "us,
Bean" spray painted in white on the split-rail
fence down the road from the old, ochre carriage
house where I live.

He fishes my red Chevy pick-up from the slick
snow when I land it in a ditch. We plan to read
everything together, and he lets Annie run him
down the Monon Trail.

In one of his poems, he writes about needing both a motorcycle and a gun. I understand what this means.

This love: it feels as surreal as eating cotton candy and as natural as air.

Death of a Dog

Annie has a cancerous growth on her side, which the vet easily removes. I supplement her diet with spices like turmeric, which I read has healing properties. But the cancer spreads to the base of her tail. We are faced with a tough decision. She's a coonhound, likes to point with her tail when she hunts. We have it removed, and she has phantom pain.

My vet helps me order her a bed with magnets inside, a palliative measure.

That spring, Rick and I take Annie with us on a road trip to Florida. On the beach in the sun, with the wind in her ears, it's like she isn't sick at all.

By summer's end, I am walking with Annie when an elderly neighbor shakes his head and says, "How long are you going to let her go on like that?" The vet tells me Annie will let me know when it is time.

In September, I see the resignation in her bloodshot eyes and sense she's over this life. I pet her for what will be the last time in our living room while our vet waits in the kitchen. Rick is at my side at first, then it's just me and my coonhound.

I've had Annie for a long time, and it hasn't been perfect. She was never properly housebroken, and when I'd stay with Dad and Jan, she'd shit in their basement.

One time when I was down to my last ten dollars, I bought some chicken wings and fries, then ran back in the restaurant to get some ketchup. By the time I got back to the car, Annie had eaten all of my carry-out food.

And yet Annie has been a constant in my life for the past several years. A faithful companion, she's never happier than when I come home.

When I'm finished saying goodbye, the vet and I switch rooms, and I cry like I don't think I've ever cried before as Shotgun Annie takes her last road trip in the trunk of his car.

Later that night, I listen to "The Weight" by The

Band over and over again. I'd always sing her
that song, thinking it was about someone named
"Annie," not "Fannie."

I don't care, it's still our song.

Take a load off Annie,
Take a load for free.

Waiting for the Sun

When winter hits, I get more depressed than
usual. February's gunmetal sky goes on forever.

I can go to work, but while I'm there, it feels
like I'm acting in a play. By the evenings, I'm
zapped, wondering how I can go in for the next
day's performance.

It seems in addition to manic depression, which
by now is called bipolar disorder, my doctor
says I may have seasonal affective disorder
(SAD). I sit under a special lamp with fake rays
from the sun and wait for spring.

The Promise

Rick is ok with me having bipolar disorder.
I give him the memoir by Patty Duke Astin.

After reading it, he makes me promise never to leave him.

Toddlers in Arms

Rick and I get married shortly after his divorce is final. My only regret is destroying a family.

Within two years, we adopt two toddler boys from Ethiopia. Holding them in my arms brings a joy I have never known.

Things I Love about Our Boys

The way they light up when they see food or me.

Their laughter, like chimes. Their peaceful faces in sleep. And the way they love Rick, calling him "Pop" from the very first day.

My Headbangin' Ethiopian Sons

On the way to pick up a prescription for tapeworm medication, I notice my sons in the backseat flailing their arms and singing word for word the lyrics to Bruce Springsteen's "Born in the U.S.A."

They can't even speak English yet.

But they can sing it. From that moment on, music becomes our bridge.

Army Pants

It doesn't take the boys long to lose their Amharic language and develop a penchant for chicken fingers. Yakob acquires a sweet tooth. Ayalkbet enjoys classic rock.

They both fall in love with superheroes like Batman, Spiderman, and the Power Rangers. Through these characters, they learn their first lessons of good versus evil.

When September 11 comes, it is all but impossible to shield our sons from the news. Soon, their Lego inventions become implements of war.

One night, we're out to dinner. Eight men in army fatigues walk in and sit at a table behind us. The boys stare, gawk, and wave. It is like Superman and the members of the entire Justice League are dining at the next table. When we finish eating, the boys circle the men's table blowing at them with straws in their mouths. Yakob asks, "Are you going to get the bad men?" "We're going to make sure everyone's safe," says one soldier.

On the way home, Yakob blurts, "Army pants can't die!" Ayalkbet explains to him that they're not army *pants*. They are army *men*. They *wear* pants, he says.

Morally, I feel like I should explain that army pants can die. That many army pants have died in many wars. But I don't.

Joy and Sorrow

Even with all this joy, tears surface.
Sometimes, I feel too much like when I listen to John Denver sing "How the life in the mountains is living in danger. From too many people, too many machines."

Things That Make Me Happy

Color. Sunshine on my face.
Puppy breath. A hot drink
on a cold day.

A blanket of snow. A forest of trees.
Clear lakes and streams.
Music and writing.

Things That Make Me Sad

Roadkill. Racism.

Starving people.
Power-drunk politicians.

The elderly crying out like babies.
Stray dogs and cats.
Motherless children.

Black Dog

Nellie is a stray dog, a springer spaniel mix
with a head shaped like a pit bull and a deep,
demonic bark. She came to our front door the
same week Annie died. I took it as a sign she
was meant to be with us. Plus, how could I
turn her away? We could count her ribs jutting
out beneath mangy, black fur. We already have
Bear, a border collie–German shepherd mix, and
Dude, a Jack Russell terrier.

But when I'm feeling well, I have a tendency to
take on more, like I'm making up for something.

Bloomington

Our family of four plus our three dogs move
to Bloomington, where I went to college and
where Rick is going to get his master's in
education.

Bloomington has a good vibe. The town takes

care of both its people and its trees…and it feels more like home to me than Noblesville, where I'm from.

The Drive-through Zoo

On a vacation out west somewhere in Missouri, we see a sign for an exotic and wild animal zoo. I plead with Rick to stop at the roadside attraction.

But Rick likes to make good time on trips. He protests my request, but I tell him it'll be fun for the kids. Soon after pulling in we're in bumper-to-bumper traffic, following behind a family in a mini-van feeding the ostriches.

Nellie and Bear are barking in the back of the Dodge truck with a king cab. I can feel the vehicle shaking when they take their excitement up a notch as they see buffalo.

Traffic is moving painstakingly slow, like the time spent waiting for the results of an x-ray. While we're in stopped traffic, Rick gets in back to calm the dogs who continue to snarl and hurl themselves against the window, and I take the wheel. The boys are wide-eyed and quiet as we move through a herd of antelope.

The kids in the car in front of us are feeding every zoo habitant in sight. Rick is leaning against the window holding onto a dog with each hand. "I think I'm having a heart attack," he says as we pass a dark green pond with no signs of life in it.

Nearly two hours later, we have seen every kind of animal except polar bears.

Rick is as sulky as the hot, bored tigers in their cage at the end of the exhibit.

When I pull over at the gas station, he is still angry with me.

Later, I spy a sign for the "World's Largest Prairie Dog." I focus my attention on the expanse of farmland and don't say a word.

Cleaning

While the boys are at preschool, I feel pressure to get things done, like cleaning and writing. We all know which is more fun.

And yet I try to take good care of our home, rubbing lemon oil into our butcher block countertops, making them shine before polishing my words.

Part of being an adult is doing the right thing, even when you don't want to.

When I'm Eighty-Four

I now work for a company that provides non-medical care to seniors.

When I first meet Bernice, she isn't wearing her dentures. She gives me a tour of her home, then I help her with a bath. She sits on a beige, plastic shower chair. I hand her towels, dry her feet.

Next, I clean her bathroom, make her bed, and dust the sunroom, while she sits at the kitchen table shuffling through the newspaper.

Meals on Wheels is bringing her lunch.
"I bet they're bringing carrots," she says.
Her eyes are bright. She likes carrots.

Sitting next to her while she eats, I can tell she likes the company. She makes little slurping noises as her tongue hits her dentures. I tell her about my family, she tells me she has two daughters. We decide Friday we'll go to the grocery store.

Later at home, as I'm brushing my teeth, I

wonder what I'll be like when I'm eighty-four and if our sons will live nearby. Rick teases that they'll have to change our diapers one day. But it isn't so funny to me.

Rascal

Today I see a dead raccoon in the road.

It wears a grimace and has a rib poking up through its belly. It makes me think how when I was a kid, we had a tame, orphaned baby raccoon named Rascal.

Mom gave him rides on the tractor.
Once, after a ride she set him down, but he ran back for more and got mangled in the blade before she could cut the engine.

Brains on Display

I'm writing a story about a medical museum on the grounds of the now-closed Central State Hospital.

The museum was once a state-of-the-art medical research and teaching facility.

There are rows and rows of jars filled with the brains of former Central State patients.

They are swimming in liquid in their amber-colored enclosures. The brains themselves are the color of canned, halved mushrooms.

I can't help but think how if I'd been alive in the late 1800s, one of those brains would be mine.

Country Comfort

Rick says Nellie is like the Michael Jordan of dogs. The problem is she uses her energy in the wrong ways, kind of like me when I'm manic.

I can't walk her without a prong collar.
She has bitten two dogs in our neighborhood and is becoming increasingly aggressive with Dude.

Rick finds her a farm to live on way out in the country in Brown County. He recounts the story of how she hopped out of his truck and ran around with her new owner as he showed her the barns.

We keep in touch with the country couple for a while, taking comfort in the fact that they love her and she's happy and that her new mom gives her flea powder each night and keeps bows in her hair.

Sometimes loving an animal means setting it free.

Tea and Tears

I arrive at the Mother's Day tea almost five minutes late, because I'm always trying to do one more thing.

The children are lined up ready to sing. Ayalkbet's voice is as pure and true as his deep belly laughs. As I gaze at my son singing to me, I realize that if you can be swallowed up by love and reverence, I am in this moment.

His teacher has to nudge me forward, so he can give me a flower. As I take it, I know he doesn't understand my tears.

A Bug's Life

On a trip to North Carolina, one of the largest dragonflies I have ever seen smacks our windshield. It is like a tiny helicopter coming in for a crash landing. The impact tears its enormous wings, giving them the jagged crosshatch design of a broken porch screen.

I watch the dragonfly's legs move slightly and wonder if it was the wind or the last evidence of life. Rick turns on the wipers, but the insect stays wedged between the windshield and the right wiper for the remainder of the trip. Rick keeps saying, "Don't look at it." Our sons are oblivious, sitting in the backseat playing with their Game Boys.

When we get to Wilmington, our destination, I ask Rick to pull into a subdivision. I slowly pluck the insect from the windshield, half-hoping it is still alive, vainly wishing that it survived not only the crash but also the two-hour trip at 70 mph.

I lay the dead dragonfly in the yard and examine it. The coloring is a gorgeous dark metallic green—a color I've seen before on fancy cars.

His legs curl in finality. My husband interrupts me, calling out the window, "Come on, you're embarrassing me."

-SIX-

Wiping the Slate Clean

I see a new doctor in 2002 who promises a
holistic approach. I tell him about my history
and how I sometimes get depressed, but that I
haven't been manic since 1988.

He tells me he's willing to wipe the slate clean,
"to see what we're really dealing with,"
and takes me off meds.

Laughter

I'm teaching an exhibit marketing class for a
week. It's eight hours each day plus a commute
to Indy. I get up at 4:30 a.m. to prepare and
drink lots of coffee and smoke lots of cigarettes.

By the end of the week I am laughing in class
so hard that I spit water.

Only I don't know what is so funny.

Dinner with Doppelgangers

We go to dinner at a Greek restaurant
called The Trojan Horse.

Tucked in a booth with Rick I peer around
and begin to notice everyone in the restaurant
is someone I know. There are a lot of former
coworkers from when Rick ran a company.
Mick and Kathie are sitting together. So are
Keith and Randy. I wait in anticipation for my
surprise dinner to begin. I don't mention to Rick
that I know about the impending festivities or
that some people are already here.

When the party never begins I figure the people
from my past will meet us at the house.

Outside the restaurant thick, wet snowflakes
twirl down to the ground. It's like walking
inside a snow globe.

Rocks

I tell our boys we should paint some rocks.
We collect them outside and bring them to the
sweet, little, white-tiled table in our kitchen.

As we paint I discover I can swirl colors together, creating patterns like on a tie-dyed shirt. The boys do it too, and soon paint drips into the grout of the table forever staining it with markings of mania.

An Offering

The next day while Rick is at work I call up the contractor who helped us remodel our house last year and announce that we need to read Tom Robbins' *Still Life with Woodpecker* together. When Rick finds out he's afraid I am getting manic. He takes me to see my therapist, to get her opinion on whether I should be hospitalized. In her office I can't sit still. I produce a white plastic bag filled with random things—CDs, return address labels, a newspaper, and a children's book.

I think the objects are proof I have reached enlightenment and hand each one to her like an offering.

Parallel Lives

She recommends waiting a few days to see if things get better. They don't. When I get the notion of parallel lives I put on my black velvet bathrobe I bought for our wedding night as a funeral shroud. I think Rick is dead, that I should wear it to mark the end of our relationship in this lifetime. I know we'll be together as soulmates again, but I am still angry he has died.

Rick is becoming his favorite singer, John Mellencamp, in one life and getting back together with his ex-wife in another.
In reality, he is busy sweeping up the colorful fragments of the Fiestaware I throw against the wall. Later I don't recall doing this. It's a detail Rick fills in for me. I just remember bits and pieces like loose beads I catch and string together.

In my parallel life, I am looking for the cowboy who would take me in his Winnebago to Madison, Wisconsin, to be part of a six-person think tank led by the writer Lorrie Moore to save the environment. Before I can go on my trip, I must vacuum and put on the coffee.

Rick yanks the vacuum's cord from the socket hissing, "Dammit, you'll wake up the boys!"

Winter's Embrace

Dude, our Jack Russell, benefits from my psychosis because I keep opening the garage door and running outside into winter's embrace.

He thinks it's a game and bolts into the night.
Now Rick has to catch his manic wife, and his
manic dog, too.

Set Me Free

At the hospital when I see the other patients and
staff, I raise my hand, move it back and forth
offering blessings to everyone while intoning,
"Set me free. Set me free. Set me free."

I spy my stepdad vacuuming the hall, then my
dad and Jerry Garcia working at the nurses'
station.

Later I stand motionless underneath the
television that is bolted to the wall. I am waiting
to get sucked into it.

The Assassin

They take me outside for cigarettes with another
patient. I think the attendant is Dr. Martin
Luther King, Jr. and the patient with the bright
red hair is the man who will kill him.

As the technician lights the man's cigarette
the shot goes off. A flutter of birds rises from

the bushes. "No! No!" I cry out. The attendant reassures me he isn't dead, tells me to look into his eyes.

"Who do you see?" he asks. I look into his dark brown eyes.

"My son," I say. "I see Yakob."

Visiting Hours

Rick visits me in the hospital. We are in the cafeteria. I turn to the pale patient next to me, who is sitting quietly, and introduce him to Rick as my husband.

Mania's Twin

When the Seroquel sets in and my thoughts are no longer flying faster than my tongue can speak them, I am released.

The problem is, in short order, depression, mania's fraternal twin, steps in to take over.

Prayer for Mom

This depression is crippling.

Michele drives up from Dallas, Georgia, where

she now lives, and cleans our bathroom because I can't.

At dinner one night, Yakob prays, "Thank you for this day, thank you for this food. And help Mom not be sad anymore."

Fighter Girl

My doctor increases my anti-depressant, I get a life coach, read self-help books, write about what I'm feeling, take vitamin supplements, try Reiki energy healing, anything to get better…

I have minimal results, but at least I am aware that there is more than one way to fight.
At least I am trying.

In a Fog

One winter morning while everyone is gone, sadness engulfs me. I feel despair akin to that which hangs in the air at the saddest of nursing homes, and I decide to go for a drive.

The fog sits low in the sky as I head toward Lake Monroe. I find the place where we go to swim in the summer. The parking lot and ice on the lake are covered with snow. I feel a crunching under my tires and wonder if I've

accidentally driven onto the ice.
Panic floods me, and I turn the car around. At
least I know I don't want to die.

Bored Cousin

The depression lingers on through most of
spring. Although I'm able to distract myself,
it's always there to some degree, following me
around like a bored cousin at a boring family
reunion. Then, more and more, it begins to leave
me alone, until one day, I realize I don't notice it
anymore.

-SEVEN-

Chickens

We live in Bloomington for three years before moving to Wilmington, North Carolina, where Rick lands a dream teaching job. We target Wilmington because it's got a milder climate, more days of sunshine, the ocean. And it's not as far away as some of the other places we've considered like Santa Fe or Sedona. Wilmington is also a river town and a college town steeped in history.

Our new house comes with chickens. After talking to Phil, the former owner, Rick decides to keep them, naming them Henny and Penny.

"He did say to watch for rats," says Rick. "Great," I mutter. We discover the rats are attracted to the chickens' food because when Rick takes the lid off the metal food container,

they converge in the pen. Rick has to bang the
lid to make them scatter.

In October, a hurricane comes our way.
The sky takes on an eerie, greenish-grey cast.
Outside, it sounds like an industrial vacuum
cleaner. We lose power for nine hours, just long
enough to spoil our food.

The next day looks like a wasteland, with fallen
limbs everywhere. There is silence except for
the chainsaws buzzing from the homes where
trees are down.

As we assess the damages, Bear bounds over to
us, depositing a dead baby squirrel at our feet.
Having fallen from a nest the small, nearly
translucent rodent is a casualty of the storm.

Other things happen. Our home is almost
broken into by muscled men, one with thick
metal chains adorning a tattooed chest.

I manage to run to a neighbor's house.
The police want to know more, say my
description fits with other recent incidents.

I total my Subaru Forester in the burgeoning
traffic swelling with tourists. The boys are in
the backseat when our Subaru spins. My airbag

deploys. Blood pours from Yakob's mouth.
His eyes are wide with shock, bits of glass and
blood in his hair.

Ayalkbet cries softly, but looks unhurt.

In what seems like seconds, there's a wail of
sirens. Every voice sounds like it comes from a
faraway cavern. The EMTs load Yakob onto a
yellow board. "We're going lights and sirens,"
one of them says.

The doctor orders a full-body MRI. Luckily, his
injuries are superficial. But I am broken.

In June, I give the last of Henny and Penny's
eggs to the neighbors, along with everything
else in the fridge.

Rick says we're doing the right thing by leaving.
"You don't know this, but at night, while you
were sleeping, the rats would come up on our
front porch."
"They did?" I ask. "What did they look like?"
"They were big," he says with a sigh, as he turns
down the busy road behind our former home.
"Just very big."

And yet I feel as though I'm betraying
something by leaving. Wilmington is a beautiful

city, it just isn't right for us. It just isn't right for me.

Aiken

A book about best college towns to retire in lists Aiken, South Carolina, as an option.

It is actually a little bit closer to Bloomington than Wilmington and offers just as much sun. No more fake sun for me. You can get to the ocean and back on a day-trip.

Rick finds a teaching job at the high school, so we buy a Cape Cod with a pool on a couple of wooded acres and settle in.

I am hopeful this adventure will be our last.

The Caterpillar Cue

I am riding shotgun in Rick's van with the window open when a butterfly bounces off the roof and lands on my leg, leaving a trail of pale, yellow mucus. I squirm at the sight and pick up the dead insect. In the split second I hold it before flinging it out the window, I can feel its brown and orange wings are warm and soft like velvet.

I feel rattled by its death, and stressed. In addition to getting acclimated, I have yet to find a job. We are doing some remodeling, plus the kids will be starting school soon. I sigh...so much to do.

Later that day, at the local art center where I pick up the boys from a class, I notice some wooden ornaments carved into the shape of butterflies. There is also a painting of a butterfly, its wings unfolding in a spray of colors. I realize I've seen more butterflies during these first weeks in Aiken than I've seen in my whole life.

Some are as big as birds. I'd see them on flowers, or flitting above my head by our swimming pool, or bobbing in the tall grass alongside the road. I'd watch them dart across the yard, eluding Maggie, our golden retriever mix.

At home, I pull out *Animal Speak* by Ted Andrews to learn that the butterfly teaches us not to fear change, but to embrace joy instead.

With the sunnier days and milder climate, conditions in Aiken are conducive to butterfly life. Temperatures impact the length of each stage of the insect's life cycle—egg to caterpillar/larva to pupa/chrysalis to the adult butterfly.

It seems the butterflies are appearing in full force, reminding me of the possibility of a graceful transition.

Rusty's Lesson Number One

I notice an ad placed by a local animal rescue in the newspaper, spotlighting a small, blind rat terrier named Rusty, who was found by the side of the road. I decide we have to adopt him.

He spends the first few days memorizing the house, like he's on an adventure. When he bangs his head into the wall while learning his way, he jumps back and sputters, "Sshoo!" then gives a little shrug and moves on.

If only hitting bumps in the road were always this easy.

Small Talk

With the kids in school, I volunteer for hospice, because I need to help. The stench of urine and bleach hits me as I enter the nursing home. I'm trying to make a small difference in the last leg of Rosalyn's journey. I search the breakfast cart for her tray.

In her room, she lies curled in a fetal position, her eyes vacant. A pile of white hair is gathered in a ponytail at the top of her head. Weighing all of eighty pounds, she has bedsores and her little hands are contracted.

Two aides hoist her up and prop some pillows behind her head. They work in unison and don't speak to Rosalyn as they mold her into an upright position. When they leave, I ask her if she's hungry, but Rosalyn is non-verbal. I lift the plastic lid covering her meal. Two mixtures of pureed food lie in round globs on the plate. One is the color of oatmeal, the other gray.

After raising the spoon to her mouth, I watch as some of the food dribbles down her chin. I wipe it off. After two more spoonfuls I think she might be thirsty. "Are you ready for a drink?" I ask before placing the straw from the carton of milk to her lips.

Designing Women is on the TV. I can hear the clatter of trays down the hall. Rosalyn belches. It takes me forty-five minutes to feed her.

She looks so tiny, her thin shoulders jutting out like chicken wings. Rosalyn wears a patch that releases pain medication. I wonder how her caretakers know how much to give her if she can't talk.

On the wall by the window, there is a small bulletin board with cards addressed to "grandma" and various pictures of adults and children. "Are these your children and grandchildren?" I ask.

Rosalyn attempts to speak, making guttural noises. Her eyes widen. But the conversation can go no further, and I'm left to wonder about the life she had before it was reduced to pain patches and pureed food.

That night at dinner, I light candles. As we make small talk, I study the faces of my family, aglow in the light.

Abilify

I find a new job at an assisted living home as an activity assistant. Now it's time to find a new psychiatrist. I have trouble locating a good one and need more meds, so I travel to the coast upon a coworker's recommendation, to meet with a new doctor.

The first thing he does is take my picture, which I think is weird. Then for the next hour he documents my history, keying it into his laptop, which also makes me uncomfortable. He says it doesn't sound as much like bipolar as it does post-traumatic stress disorder, and he wants to change my meds.

But I've been down that road before.
For the past few years, I've been taking Abilify, which seems like a clean drug with minimal side effects. With Abilify I don't have to get my blood drawn.

Plus, on some level, I buy into the marketing of my current medication with its implied promise to "abilify" you, to make you achieve all your dreams.

One problem with Abilify, which is considered part of a new class of anti-psychotic medication, is no one knows the long-term effects.
I guess one day, I will.

I'm not going back to the new doctor. I figure I may very well have PTSD, as he suggested, but for now, I'm doing my best to manage bipolar disorder.

Hello, Hoa

I'm becoming friends with one of the neighbors, who early on decides she will cut the boys' hair

and that she'd like her sons to come over for
swims in our pool.

She's got opinions on everything from what
color of paint we've selected for the kitchen
to the quantity of dogs we own. She likes to
counsel me on things like being thrifty, which
goes in one ear and out the other, like the words
of a bossy, older sister.

And yet making new friends at this age isn't
easy. I'll take what I can get.

Parenting

Time flies when you're a parent.
And there are no do-overs.

If Dogs Could Talk

Life would be easier if our four dogs could talk.
Bear could answer why, after eight years of no
accidents in the house, he suddenly decides to
take regular dumps in our dining room.

I would also like to know the reason why
Maggie, our golden retriever–Chow mix
whom we adopted in Wilmington, stares at me
sometimes. She doesn't shift her gaze unless I
distract her attention.

Dude is the best communicator. I can figure out his demands from the tone of his barks: the growly one says, "Get me my damn ball, woman. It's under the couch again." The high-pitched staccato says, "Are you crazy? Let me in. It's cold out here!"

Rusty, the newest member of our canine club, is also expressive. He yips when he's hungry, or doesn't want to be alone, or hears the laughter of children through the fence and wants to join in.

At the dog bakery, they're having a fundraiser where you can talk to an animal communicator for a donation.

When we meet the communicator, Rick is skeptical, but the boys seem mesmerized by the woman. She has shiny, dark hair with streaks of gray framing her face and protruding eyes that glisten like obsidian. She speaks with a dramatic flair, moving her hands like she's catching butterflies.

"Tell me about your pets," she says. "What are their names?" I tell her all of our dogs' names. "What kind of dog is Bear?" she asks, making slow eye contact with each of us.

Rick tells her he's a border collie–German shepherd mix. "We call him 'freight train' because he's so big," adds Yakob.

"What about the other ones?" she asks.

Yakob describes the breeds.

"It's like this," she says with certainty. "Bear is the CEO. He really wants you to know that he's big and strong. I can't say enough how important this is."

She inhales deeply, closing her eyes for a minute, getting a visual of our dogs. "Dude is like the sheriff. He thinks he's in charge, but Bear is definitely CEO." Rick and I glance at each other. Dude *is* like a sheriff.

"Who is the one with digestive problems?" asks the communicator. "Maggie is," I blurt.

And so it goes. Rick is still dubious, especially after she says that Maggie has parasites and we should give her a mixture of hydrogen peroxide and water on the next full moon.

She also tells us Maggie is an old soul. "A healer and a shaman." I think about how Maggie looks at me. "And as for 'Rusty,' was it? He loves to play with balls."

"He's blind," Rick states. "Dude likes balls though," I add, hopefully.

"Aah. Dude is being territorial," she says, smiling. "Here he is again."

Until now I hadn't put it together that she is channeling our dogs.

She tells us Rusty has not been with us long enough to come through strongly. "My advice is to assure him that he's going to stay with you. He's a little unsure of himself. Let him know this is his forever home. Oh, and Dude says don't put him in the closet again. He doesn't like that."

Rick looks at me in surprise. As a terrorizing puppy, Dude would bite. Someone suggested putting him in a small, dark place like a closet when he did that. So after holding him down and shouting, "I'm the man of the house, not you!" Rick would put him in the closet for a few minutes. Dude hated it.

She let us know that was the last bit of information to be imparted by handing me her business card.

On the way to the car Yakob says, "You know, I thought she was pretty good."

"Me too," says Ayalkbet.

Rick is quiet. I knew he thought that much can be intuited by virtue of knowing a dog's age, sex, and breed, but there was no way she could have guessed he used to lock Dude in the closet.

Later, I hear him telling Rusty not to worry. "This is your home, Rusty. This is your forever home."

Whiskey and Easy

There's an intersection in Aiken at the corner of Whiskey Road and Easy Street, named for two famous horses.

I don't drink whiskey anymore, but with Aiken's slow pace and plenty of sunshine, I sometimes feel like the livin' is easy.

EIGHT

Holding Hands

We're at the podiatrist's office where I'm getting my calluses scraped. Rick and the boys are with me because we're going to dinner after the appointment. We've been waiting for my turn for a while and Rick starts to nod off.

A woman with a wide smile and a gold tooth walks in with a man, probably in his sixties, on her arm. She gently sets him in a chair next to Ayalkbet, who is thumbing through a *Highlights* magazine, pen in hand. His caregiver goes to the back of the office, I assume to the examination room.

The man lifts Ayalkbet's arm and begins to tap on my son's plastic wristwatch. As he does this, he keeps his eyes turned upward, straight into space. They have a deep, glassy sheen to them.

My son glances at me and smiles the sort of smile you do when a baby does something cute.

As I watch, he takes the pen from Ayalkbet and drops it into the fold of the magazine. Then he takes my son's left hand. Yakob catches my eye and raises his eyebrows.

Patients come and go. The glassy-eyed man looks up and taps his fingers against his thumbs like he is playing the flute.

This is awkward. Nervous and inappropriate laughter rises up in my chest, threatening to spew forth.

The man continues to grab his hand and pen at random. Ayalkbet calmly lets him, passing no judgment. As I watch my son, my inner turmoil subsides. As I watch my son, I realize he is one of my greatest teachers.

Death of the Sea-Monkeys

Sea-Monkeys don't really resemble the creatures in their advertisements which promise smiling mermaid-like animals. Yet when in good health they are cute, sporting little black eyes at the tops of their heads, fins, and tadpole-like tails. The males have two little curling structures on the tops of their heads like dual pompadours.

Yakob's Sea-Monkeys aren't doing so well.
Many have died. The rest are dying.

I hope to bond with my son over the small
simians. I want to share with him some of
the same fun I had as a child. Or perhaps I
am trying to relive my own childhood by
purchasing these aquatic pets.

Regardless, when the last one perishes, I want
a shot at Sea-Monkey redemption. According
to the website, when Sea-Monkeys die, you can
aerate the little plastic tank with the removable
blue lid for a week and a half, and the eggs
remaining in the bottom will hatch into babies.

I try this for several days. When I make the air
bubbles by depressing the pump at the end of
the plastic tubing and injecting the other end in
the water, it creates a tsunami of small bits of
dead Sea-Monkeys and algae. When the morbid
concoction settles, there are no signs of life.

The day of my final attempt, one of the male
carcasses does a backwards dive and lands next
to a pair of tiny, plastic green sandals. Its little
black eyes shimmer like tiny caviar. The hybrid
brine shrimp's pompadours are jagged like he'd

been in a fight.

Across the ruins, a fake Sea-Monkey lies on
a beach towel with his arms behind his algae-
shrouded head, smiling up at me just like the ad
in the comic book.

Soon after the attempts of my resuscitation fail,
Yakob comes home carrying a goldfish with a
crooked tail that he won at a church fair. He is
grinning, clutching a plastic baggie containing
the fish. "Mom, look what we got. His name is
Carter!"

When Carter dies, there are two more
replacements, also named Carter, before we give
up on aquatic pets.

Coincidence

I'm noticing a lot of coincidences lately.
I see the number 333 everywhere and notice the
clocks at 3:33.

Today, I see it on a license plate.
But I know to dwell in synchronicity could lead
me down a path I don't want to go.

It's ironic how being present and really noticing
things, which is actually healthy, when done in

extreme, can become a curse.

Sunshine in Her Soul

At the assisted living home Ms. Robar, a new resident, attends most activities. I learn that she lived with her brother before moving in, and she used to be a social worker. She wears a cross on a simple chain and often says, "I love you. God bless you."

She loves coffee and enjoys going to the little café down the street. One day, when I go to get Ms. Robar for the trip, I find her lying in bed crying. Her eyelids are red, her hair in disarray. "My brother's cat died," she says.

"I'm sorry," I say.
"*I'm* sorry for crying so much."
"That's okay. It's sad."
"The doctor said he needs to adjust my medication. I have bipolar disorder," she confesses.
"You take care of yourself," I reply. "Maybe we can get coffee next Thursday."
"Oh, I'd like that," she says. "Will you pray for my brother?"
"I'll pray for both of you," I tell her, as I notice the framed picture of a Calico cat on her bedside table.

I hesitate before leaving. I want to let her know I have bipolar disorder too, but Ms. Robar likes to talk, and soon all of the residents and staff would know.

Instead, I say, "I was really sad when my dog died."
"Oh, God bless you," she says.

The following week, Ms. Robar is feeling better and we go for coffee. Steam rises from our mugs and Ms. Robar recalls a time when she was manic. "I had to go to the hospital. I told everyone there I loved the sunshine in their souls."

I take a sip of my coffee. The times I have been manic I usually recognize the light in everyone too.

But I hold my tongue.

Uniquely Lovely

On a trip back to Bloomington, Yakob and Ayalkbet are hammering open geodes. Yakob gets a rock stuck in his hand. When we get home, I take him to the doctor, who says the foreign body is embedded in a growth plate.

To remove the dirty object requires surgery with full anesthesia. During the procedure, I am edgy. Outside the building I take big breaths, look up at the sky and begin to bargain with God. Later in the recovery room, I kiss Yakob. He smiles, curling in his bottom lip as he always does.

A nurse reviews his prescription instructions with us, and I head to the drug store, elated that the procedure is over. While waiting for the medications, I wonder how in the world a rock made it through that little cut deep into his bone.

Not only that, but the rock was part of a geode, a natural gift which is uniquely lovely and light-filled, like my son.

On the way home, Yakob wants to stop at his school to show off his wound.

If he continues to keep his spirit, I'll know we've done a good job raising him.

Lucky

My friend Kay from Indiana calls. She's on a cross-country journey and wants to visit. Kay holds a crucial piece to the boys' histories. She, along with my brother Todd, brought them home from Ethiopia for us. While sitting around a bonfire in the backyard, she recounts the stories.

"On the plane ride home, you kept shoving crackers in your mouth," she tells Ayalkbet. "I'd put one in my mouth and chew slowly to show you how, but you kept doing it."

Ayalkbet laughs.

"And you just slept through it," she says to Yakob. He smiles and fixes himself a second s'more.

As I watch my sons enjoy the stories of their humble beginnings, I feel lucky to be their mom. But then I have a reoccurring thought. We are almost half way through raising them, and time is running out. When all is said and done, will they feel lucky too?

Anxiety to Boot

Having dealt with my illness mostly successfully for eighteen years, I get leveled with another blow: panic attacks. Ever since we were nearly broken into, I started getting anxious about being home alone. Over time, it gets worse. I share some of my feelings with Hoa. She also knows I have bipolar.

Hoa and I go to yard sales and sometimes sit on the back porch to paint our nails.

One day, she drives me to a yard sale out in the country. I become anxious as I lose my bearings. Hoa says this yard sale is inside.

I survey the tiny duplex on the scrubby plot of land and grow suspicious. It feels like there's an elephant sitting on my chest. I tell her I'll wait in the car.

When she ducks inside, I leave a voicemail for Rick doing my best to describe where I am in case I don't make it home.

The Perfect Storm

Rick likes to keep things neat and orderly. He keeps his car much tidier than mine and can't stand clutter. He also likes his Jack Russell to be as clean as possible which is no small feat since Dude enjoys digging and rolling in animal carcasses and droppings, when they are available.

We've had Dude, a handsome, tri-colored Jack, since he was a puppy. He came from a litter belonging to Kay who has always had Jack Russells. He's the only pure-bred we've ever owned, and although Kay didn't give us any papers, Rick likes to say of the dog, "He's got f-ing papers," like John Goodman's line in *The Big Lebowski*. Our dog is in fact named after Jeff Bridges' character in the same movie.

From the get-go, Dude bonded with Rick. He's a man's dog, and when he was a pup, Rick would whistle "Strangers in the Night" into his ear at bedtime until Dude started crooning along with him. In addition to having selective listening, our now mature Dude has a few other quirks, among them a fear of water and a hatred of thunderstorms.

As with most homes, there are things that must be done for maintenance. Rick insists on replacing the gutters with the kind that have a covering that keeps debris out.

When the workers leave, I let Dude and Maggie out onto the deck. Even though the skies threaten an impending storm, they've been in all day. Bear elects to stay inside because he knows I'll be cooking dinner soon and Rusty is asleep. Rick appears in the kitchen, and I warn him that it looks like rain and to bring the dogs in.

"There's time," he replies. "It's their favorite part of the day, and they haven't run yet."

"If it storms, you won't be able to catch Dude,"
I say.

While Rick is out back with Maggie and Dude,
I hear a rumbling of thunder and step onto the
deck to assist with getting the dogs. Maggie
is obedient, rushing inside.

Dude remains at large with a shoe in his mouth
which he shakes furiously at the thunder. It
starts raining and I go inside, thinking Rick will
eventually catch him.

When I hear Rick yelling minutes later, I go
back outside. My husband is sopping wet with
sweat and rain. His grey and black hair, which
he's kept longer lately, is frizzy in the humidity.
In fact, he looks a bit like Gene Wilder. Dude is
covered in mud and has no intention of coming
inside.

"Watch him!" orders Rick. "I'm getting the
hose."
"Why?" I ask.
"Can't you see him? Can't you *smell* him?" asks
Rick. "He's rolled in shit."
I look down at Dude who's covered in tan poop
up to his neck. The dog runs toward the shed
shaking Ayalkbet's tennis shoe from
side to side as he goes.

86

"Dammit, I told you to watch him. Now he's going to roll in it some more!"

"I told YOU to bring him in earlier," I shout, heading inside and slamming the door behind me.

Several minutes later, I notice that the storm has picked up, and I go find Rick to insist he get inside, regardless of what Dude chooses to do. Rick is chasing Dude along the side of the fence, spraying at him with the hose. My husband has on his wading boots and rubber gloves. His floral shirt and Bermuda shorts top off the look.

"It's not animal shit. It's human!" he yells.

"What do you mean? Did the boys do it?" I shout into the whipping wind.

"I think it was one of the workers. There's a pile behind the shed where he's been rolling."

"How do you know it is human?" I ask.

"I'm covered in it, for one reason," he says. "I know the difference."

About an hour later, Dude gives up the fight and lets Rick hose him down. Rick brings him inside and dries the weary animal with an old towel, then locks him in the garage. From the kitchen, I hear him on the telephone down the hall in the office.

"Look," he says, "I'm just telling you what happened. I don't know who it was, but I'm telling you they went to the bathroom in our yard, and it wasn't number one, and I'm not very happy about it."

From the kitchen, I suppress giggles.
Rick's voice rises as I stir the pasta.

Close Call

I'm writing an essay about a retired sailor I used to help in college. It's the best piece I've written in a while, maybe ever.

While I'm working on our screened porch, Rick checks on me. I'm careful to cover up my overflowing ashtray, a tell-tale sign I'm overdoing it.

That night, I can't sleep, and wonder if I'm getting manic. I take a hot bath, drink some chamomile tea. Finally I get tired, sleep a solid eight.

It's a close call, but I think I've had a writer's high, not a manic one.

Goodbye, Hoa

Hoa hasn't been calling. She normally phones every morning after the kids get off to school. When I ask her what gives, she says she doesn't understand why I got scared at the yard sale the other day.

"Your schizophrenia, or whatever it is…I just can't handle it anymore."

And just like that, it's goodbye, Hoa.

Funky

Sometimes, I think I'm getting depressed, only to realize it is PMS.

Occasionally, I don't feel like doing anything but discover I'm just bored.

Other times, I get in a funk for no apparent reason. Most women have the blues on occasion. I am just extra attuned to them because if they get to a certain point, the bottom could fall out.

-NINE-

The Goodbye Girl

Aiken feels like home, but we find ourselves
unable to make ends meet. Rick decides he
needs to go back into technical sales. He strikes
a deal with the new owners of his old company.
They invite him to open an office in Franklin,
Tennessee.

Despite the packing we do, as the weeks pass,
Ayalkbet holds on to the hope that we won't go.
The worse part about moving for kids is
saying goodbye to their peers. He's friends
with our neighbors, especially the girl, Annie.

When moving day comes and the car is loaded,
he sits on the hill with her. A little later, as we
pull away from our home for the last time,
she runs alongside the car, pressing her hands
against the glass of his window. The girl's

golden, wavy ponytail bounces as she slows, giving up the chase.

Our car nears the corner of the street and Ayalkbet rolls down his window, sticking his head out to look back at her standing in the road. I can't tell if she is crying, but I am fighting tears.

When he was little, I could bandage his scraped knee, but he is older now, and I cannot fix his broken heart.

Keeping Watch

My husband, our sons, Bear, Dude, Maggie, and Rusty along with three grey tabbies we adopted while in South Carolina, make our new home in Franklin, which is about a half-hour south of Nashville and only five hours from Indiana. The landscape features rolling hills, and there's even more churches than there were in Aiken.

Franklin has a quaint and bustling downtown where country stars are often spied. In the center of the downtown square is a monument of a Confederate soldier who seems to be keeping watch over the town. Maybe he'll watch over us too.

Moving Is a Bitch

Even though we've become old pros at it,
moving is still a bitch.

Unpacking, painting, putting up a fence for the
dogs, not to mention the money we lose paying
realtors and movers.

Money causes stress. Stress causes anxiety.
Anxiety causes trouble.

Settling In

In short order, the boys make lots of new
friends, join the local travel soccer team, and
settle in their new school.

Rick gets busy building his client base, and I
start looking for a job.

Along the way, I find my favorite shops and
coffee houses.

When fall approaches, it's still milder than
Indiana. Fall is always a busy time, and in
Franklin it's no different.

I take my meds, look for work, write a bit. I try
my best at being a good mother, a good wife.

Enough

The sun's intensity is fading as if by a dimmer switch. There's a crispness in the air that only occurs this time of year.

Halloween, one of my grandmother's favorite holidays, is just around the corner. She loved arranging spooky knick-knacks which she called "do-das" and greeting children in costumes at her door. Gram savored the little things in life—a hot cup of decaf Sanka, a game of Yahtzee, Jergens hand cream, and Gerbera daisies.

When I turned 38, something about being on the far side of thirty gave me pause, and I began to take stock of my genetic heritage. I can thank my dad for a dry sense of humor. I look to my maternal side where there is other evidence of where my traits originate.

My face, which I like well enough, most resembles Gram's middle child—Aunt Jane. Gram had three other daughters: Carol (my mom), Aunt Patty, and Aunt Susan. Uncle Bobby, the baby, died shortly before I was born. I, like my mom and all of my aunts, am sensitive and have a penchant for comfort foods like pasta.

There are darker hereditary traits in the family tree. I come by anxiety and depression naturally. My mom and aunts have all been treated for one or both mental maladies. Gram herself was said to be a worrier. I never picked up on this as a child.

Instead I'd latch on to her soft hands. She'd often put one over her mouth when something surprised her. I can still taste the tanginess of the bleu cheese in her cheese balls. We loved doing crafts.

Gram learned to drive in her twenties, wouldn't traverse interstate highways, and over time, limited herself to traveling just the five blocks to the beauty shop. Eventually, she quit navigating her red and white '57 Ford Fairlane altogether, relying on her feet to take her to get her hair done.

My driving patterns have changed too. High overpasses, bridges, and mountain roads scare me. I avoid interstates most of the time.

After my grandfather died at the age of seventy-seven, Gram succumbed to the ravages of Parkinson's disease. She moved in with Mom and my stepdad. I'd come over and sit with her when I could. At one point, I read to her from

Little Women, and, being the English major that I was, posed discussion points.

"Who is your favorite character?" I asked one day. The illness had changed her voice. The answer came slowly, as if an echo from the depths of a deep canyon.
"Jo."
She died before we could finish the book.

Soon, I'll be breaking out my own Halloween do-das—wicker pumpkins with lights, the hanging ghoul that laughs and flashes red, glowing eyes when you walk by its sensor. My sons, ten and eleven, will go trick-or-treating. This year, though, I'll reflect on the simplicity with which my grandma lived her life. And try not to worry too much.

New Doctor

I like my new doctor and tell him my history. I'm not interested in adding anti-anxiety medication to my cocktail, and he's fine with that. Most of what "Big Pharma" has to offer for that is addictive anyway.

I heard Stevie Nicks wrestled with Klonopin, I have enough of a landslide to deal with.

What I Know

I learn with moving it takes about three years
for a place to feel like home to me.
Kids adapt to new environments better than
adults. It takes them about three months.

I don't know what I envy more about children,
their childlike innocence, or their resilience.

To Market, to Market

I take a job in the kitchen at a local market/deli.

It's perfect because I work ten to three. I can
write for a couple of hours once the boys are at
school and be home by the time they are done.

The kitchen is close to our house. No highway
driving required.

After a while, being on my feet five hours a day
serving up lunches at the counter, doing dishes,
and cleaning makes me feel stronger.

And I'm now pumping out around seven pages
of writing before work.

Clocking in, clocking out, I'm working like
clockwork.

Seized

Yakob calls me, saying something's wrong with
Ayalkbet. He's on the ground and won't get up.

I rush to the park, find his body in spasms, eyes
vacant.

For a minute I'm outside my body.
Looking down at him I think he's dying, my
baby son is dying, and there will never be
anything more.

Thank God it isn't death but a seizure.

In the hospital, intensive testing shows no
known cause.

The doctor tells us everyone is allowed one
seizure.

Later, I think about my own brain and wonder
how many psychotic breaks are allowed.

Be a Better...

Sometimes I get really down on myself,
thinking I want to be a better mother wife
daughter sister friend.

But then, who doesn't have these thoughts?

Family Traditions

The holidays are fast approaching. On Christmas Eve, we are starting a new tradition of exchanging pajamas to wear the next morning. I hear that Faith Hill and Tim McGraw do this with their family. It seems like a fun idea, although I'm wondering if it will stick.

During the first couple of Christmases we shared with the boys, I lit a special candle in honor of their Ethiopian mothers. While I think of these women often, especially as the boys are getting older, I'm ashamed to admit that I don't even know where that candle is now.

In examining our consistent family rituals, the list is pretty short. I bake sugar cookies with the boys every holiday season, and they decorate them. When Yakob and Ayalkbet score a goal in soccer, we celebrate with ice cream.

This year, the downward spiral of the economy illuminates what is most important in life—sharing with and loving others. Our family has grown even closer. We plan to send a compilation of our favorite songs to friends and family. It is an inexpensive project, yet makes for what we believe is a thoughtful gift.

Our house has speakers built into every room. It is not a feature we designed but was surely enjoyed by the former owners. Rick has only recently figured out how to use the technology, so it surprises me when I'm walking in from the garage and hear the opening drum beat from Bruce Springsteen's "Born in the USA." The music blares throughout the house.

I feel a shiver up my spine as I listen to Springsteen's voice, then my eyes well up with tears.

I've heard that the sense of smell is most powerful in evoking memories, but sound must be up there too. This is one of the first tunes we sang with the boys when they came from Ethiopia. Ayalkbet starts moving his head in time to the music where he sits at the kitchen table doing his homework. "Oh, yeah," he says. He remembers.

I enter the family room where Rick is sitting on the couch with his feet propped up on the coffee table. He's got a look on his face that is a mixture of pride and nostalgia. The first few songs on the CD are ones we listened to over and over when we lived in Indiana. We associate them with where we began our life as a family. Other songs in our collection are musical staples reminiscent of different places we've lived— Wilmington, Aiken, and now Franklin.

Yakob skips in and immediately begins to cut a rug. Ayalkbet gets up from his homework and joins us. A Carole King song is playing now and we shake our behinds in unison. I break out of the line to dance closer to Bear, who jumps up, placing his front paws on my chest. He likes to dance too.

I imagine there are songs that first touched the boys' hearts long ago in Ethiopia. Perhaps their mothers sang them sweet lullabies.

Listening to music might not qualify as a family tradition, but good music, like love, is something that can be passed on and has the ability to stand the test of time.

-TEN-

Take One Tablet at Bedtime, Every Night

The instructions on my Abilify
say to take one tablet, every day.

Normally I take my 10 mg faithfully,
but lately I've been busy, forgetful even,
skipping a dose here and there.

That's ok, right?

Perennial Itch

I get the perennial itch. I want something better
than my job at the market. Something more than
a part-time job. I apply for a marketing position
at a local cat shelter.

The director, named Kat, likes me at the
interview. She tells me to jot down some ideas.

I come up with ten single-spaced pages. When I share them with Rick, he's afraid that I'm doing too much.

I assure him I've just finally gotten my creative spark back.

The Floodgates Open

I'm on to something with my writing, and I've got a fascination with Barack Obama, CSI, and cats.

When I bring my interests together on the page, I create a glorious essay I'm sure is worthy of a prize.

Bible Thumper

While my writing (mind) takes off
so does my research into the Bible.

On my desk are a Catholic version, a toddler one, which is easier to read, and a book called *Bad Girls of the Bible*.

I'm intrigued by the "woman at the well" because she doesn't have a name and she guards the water.

Shopping

The bookstore is electric. It feels like all the
books are calling for me, but I'm on the hunt for
a children's anthology called *Free to Be...You
and Me*. Locating it, I grab all five copies and
order some more.

A coffee table–sized book called *Cosmos*
catches my eye because "Cosmos," in reference
to the flower, is one of my nicknames. Then
I spy a novel called *Last Night at the Lobster*
by someone named Stewart O'Nan. The cover
looks like a scene from Indiana University.
Thumbing through it I notice two characters
have the same names as people
I work with at the market.

And then I have a knowing feeling.

My former graduate school professor, Bill,
has written a book about me under a pen name.

The Reader

At home I call Susan, whom I talk to most
nights, read to her from *Free to Be...You and
Me* with fervor. As if within its pages lies the Da
Vinci Code.

The Whisper

Rick sits on the couch as I pace around it.

"Who am I?" he asks.
"Rick," I say.
"How do you know?"
"Because you're my husband."

His next question comes as a sad whisper, "How do I know you won't forget it?"

Pregnant with Prophets

My period is late. I'm craving turkey and becoming sensitive to odors.

Even though a pregnancy test is negative, I send a postcard to my dad indicating that I might be pregnant and sign it, "Obama Mama."

My toddler Bible gives me ideas for names. I've decided I'm having twins, and I like Mary and Jonah the best.

Felines and Felons

In bed I share my insights with Rick. I believe that the solution to the feral cat problem in our country is to catch them and put them in prison.

Taking care of cats will help rehabilitate the prisoners the way it's sometimes done with dogs.

Rick pulls me closer, scooping me into a tight hug.

To the Doctor

Rick takes me to my doctor, who I assume knows about the baby prophets. He dispenses new medication I can't seem to swallow. Rick feeds me the pills in applesauce.

The Lamictal causes a rash which, left unchecked, can be fatal in patients. My doc replaces it with a stronger dose of Abilify.

The rash goes away, but the mania is here to stay.

My Angels

Our pharmacy is in a grocery store.
While waiting in line for my meds I see angels.

A young Elvis is in the line, along with Johnny Cash. As we exit the store I see Rick's mom, who's been dead for a couple of years, extract a shopping cart from the pile.

She smiles at me as she hurries inside, so Rick won't see her. These are my angels, not his.

Card Party

My high school friends are coming over for dinner and games. I divide a deck of cards for euchre.

As my excitement builds over the anticipation of their arrival I scribble notes for each of them.

When it gets late and Rick tells me to go to bed I am sure they'll be over in the morning.

Flora and Fauna

My Aunt Jane drives through a winter storm to get to me, but it is too late to help.

I show her a book about wildflowers, pointing to each one, saying, "I'm going to have my own forest with all of the flowers."

Aunt Jane listens patiently, like I'm a child reading her a book.

Arm Waddle

Aunt Jane, Rick, and I ride up the elevator

of the psychiatric hospital. Also with us is the
lady who did my intake paperwork.

I point to the woman's arm and tell her she has
"a lot of arm waddle."

Rick and Aunt Jane are silent.

The Night Nurse

An attendant stays by my side that night.
I think she's the reincarnation of Susan's mom,
who died of brain cancer many years ago.

I am afraid to go to the bathroom by myself,
even though it is only a few short feet from my
bed. I ask the nurse to wait by the door.

When I wake in the morning the caretaker is
gone.

I get to my feet unsteadily; there's a glow of
light and a hum of activity at the end of the
hallway. It's the nurses' station.

I have to hold on to the wall as I move toward it,
crying out for coffee.

Fast Healer

At the height of my confusion I think there is a
bomb in the remote control for the TV.

I am in the hospital for only a few days. Dr.
Peterson says I'm a fast healer.

Under Lock and Key

Home is a prison. Rick locks the fence
around the backyard, along with the garage
fridge where we keep water, Gatorade, and beer.

I'm not allowed to drive or use technology.
When I locate my hidden Blackberry
Ayalkbet snatches it from me, saying, "Mom,
you can't have this."

I spend a lot of time on the covered back porch
listening to the airplanes overhead.
They are full of old friends waiting to land.

A Gift Basket

The house across the street is under repair. I'm
convinced the improvements are being made
because the Obamas are moving in.

I prepare a gift basket filling it with a black

and white coffee mug with cats on it, birthday candles, fruit, a small Ethiopian flag, and some earrings for the First Lady.

I open the kitchen window and burn a candle in a diffuser with some tea tree oil, figuring the scent will welcome them.

But Rick keeps closing the window, much to my annoyance.

Mama Ain't Sane

There's a saying, "If Mama ain't happy, ain't nobody happy." But what happens when Mama ain't sane?

Mad for Music

I've got music in every room, but instead of playing the same song through the house speakers, I need to listen to everything I like, so I get out my portable CD players.

Mellencamp is in the bedroom, Sheryl Crow's on the back porch, and the Dixie Chicks are in the kitchen. Rick gets irritable about me having too much music and shuts them all off.

Later when he finds me rocking out to The

Killers in the garage, Rick yanks the cord
and hurls the CD player into the driveway. It
smashes into the asphalt.

My husband has lost his lid. The lid of the CD
player is broken too.

Angels in the Snow

One thing I miss about living up north is the
snow.

When I look outside and see it falling
I rush outdoors to make snow angels.
Yakob follows me, grabs my arm, tells me I'm
not allowed to play in the front yard.

Cigarettes, Please

Aunt Jane is monitoring me while Rick plays
basketball with the boys in the school gym.

I give her some greeting cards, a bandana,
and my grandfather's bolo tie from his square
dancing days, saying, "You know who to give
these to."

I know she knows my former professor has
taken up residence in Yakob's closet.

Per Rick's orders, Aunt Jane rations my cigarettes. When I smoke my allotted four and she doesn't give me any more, I grow agitated.

My nicotine fit lands me back in the hospital.

Just another reason to quit.

-ELEVEN-

Tomorrow

When it sinks in I'm here to stay I have a fit
in my hospital room, yell "motherfucker" in
reference to my husband while kicking my desk
chair.

Then I hear Dr. Peterson at the nurses' station
say with a laugh, "Well, maybe tomorrow will
be a better day."

Fuck him too.

Undercover Patients and FBI Agents

Nurse Katy tells me not to pay too much
attention to the other patients. This is difficult,
considering Dr. Peterson has hired some of them
to work undercover to help him figure out what
makes me tick.

Abby's on my side, though. She has a burr haircut, wears long, flowing hippie-style dresses, says group is like Kindergarten.

I ask her if she knows about the professor who wrote a book about me.

"Sister, he's at a book signing in Kansas. I was just out there with my own books."

My eyes widen. She continues, "I've got two husbands too. But don't tell anybody."

I retreat to a corner table and start drawing two fish—one pink, the other blue. I fill them in with polka dots and write, "Mary & Jonah."

Abby approaches me. I hand the drawing to her. "Don't let them see this!" she hisses, shoving it under the table. Then she says, "Never use names."

I tell Abby I might be pregnant with twins. "Shh! FBI," she says, while pointing to her chest.

Rearranging Furniture

Sometimes I feel the urge to rearrange the chairs in the day room. I line up five chairs facing the wall like when I used to sit in timeout all those years ago on the adolescent ward.

But this is not about timeout: this is about disciples and prophets. One chair is for Ayalkbet (Isaiah), one chair is for Yakob (James), two are for the baby prophets, Jonah and Mary.

The last chair is for me. I am not a disciple or a prophet, I am just the coordinator of them, making sure they all have a place to sit.

Sweet Tonic

Karen and Bryanna are detoxing from something—probably meth.

To help with cravings they sneak packets of sugar from the cafeteria, mix it with water and drink the sweet tonic.

I watch, wishing I had an elixir for my demons.

Southern Rock

Kyle, one of the patients I suspect is hired by Dr. Peterson, is a dead ringer for John Mellencamp. I wonder if he is musically inclined. He has heavy bags under his eyes and chews lots of Nicorette gum.

114

One evening I sit with him at dinner and ask what kind of music he likes. "Southern rock. Same as you." Just as I'm wondering how he knows I like Southern rock he says, "We'll listen to it before we lay down together tonight."

I don't know what he's talking about, but I wonder if this means I'm supposed to be with him when we're released. If that's true, can it mean Kyle is really a reincarnation of my husband? 'Cuz as mad as I am with Rick I'm not ready to lose him.

After dinner we watch TV. For some reason it's subtitled in what looks to be Arabic. We sit quietly and watch anyway.

I Remain

Over the passing days, Abby and Kyle go home. The addicts get to go too. But I remain.

When I lament to another patient about the list of abuses Rick has done to me, like how he changed the time on all the clocks to confuse me, she writes them down, hands them to me, and I place them on my desk. Her handwriting is pretty. The words, though, are ugly.

Puzzled

Tabitha, a technician, mostly works on the
geriatric unit, but occasionally she'll sit with us.
It's a boring Sunday afternoon, and I help her
put together a puzzle of a scene from a kitchen
with a cupboard and teacups.

As we work, Tabitha tells me she does these all
the time at home while her husband watches TV.
I think of Rick and try to remember what we
like to do.

When it's time for her to leave, she says,
"Thanks for being so good," like she had heard I
could be a handful.

SORRY!

I feel like the opponent in the game SORRY!,
who just wants to get all her men home safe.

While this isn't a game, I'm starting to feel the
edges of my anger toward Rick soften. Maybe
I'm the one who should be sorry.
I throw away my list.

Harness It for Good

When my anger does subside after another week

or so, Dr. Peterson sends me home.

Before I go, he tells me I have it better than a lot of people in the hospital, and that I can have a bright future if I "harness it for good," as if my illness is a workhorse I can whip into submission.

The Luck of the Irish

But that night my loxapine, an older anti-psychotic medication often used in treating schizophrenia, can't be filled because none of the drugstores carry it. The next morning, I take a new pregnancy test, which is also negative. Still, I cling on to hope that it is wrong.

Then, in the shower, blood comes pouring down my legs. This is not how my periods normally begin—slowly and accompanied by cramps.

I am sullen on the way to a museum in Nashville where Yakob's school's art is on display. His painting is a self-portrait with words around the edges of his face. I gaze at the word "Mom."

After viewing my son's art, I peruse the gift shop which is full of Irish objects—green scarves, jewelry with green gemstones, and books on Ireland. I know it is all for me because I'm Irish. Only I'm not feeling very lucky.

Throughout the day, my blood loss is heavier, coming out in large clots.

I'm in the bathroom when Rick tries to kiss me. I refuse him.

If I've had a miscarriage, then there's also been a miscarriage of justice, and I can't be expected to kiss and make up so soon.

-TWELVE-

911

My third hospitalization involves me spitting
Doritos in Rick's face as he and the boys try
to get me in the car. An ambulance is quick to
respond to my husband's 911 call.

Betty and Don are working the night shift.
My eyes bleed tears as I tell them about my
miscarriage, pointing to the marks on my arms
and legs from Rick's effort to get me in the car.

I want to know if they have a camera to
document the abuse. They put me to bed.

We Line Up

In the hospital we line up for medication.
We line up for breakfast. We line up.

In the hospital we line up for group.
We line up for dinner. We line up.

Sometimes the lines get broken.
Charlie makes a beeline for the kitchen,
spilling soup as he goes. Code green.

Diane falls. She's having a seizure.
The line becomes a circle. Code blue.

Eliza's off by herself, crying again.
Tears ride the lines of her face.

In the hospital we line up for popcorn.
We line up for bed. Some of us sleep, some of
us can't. In the morning we line up for vitals.
We are alive.
We line up.

Loser

The good thing about persistent mania is I'm
losing weight.

The bad thing is I'm losing my sons.

White Coat

He breezes in, spends what seems like thirty
seconds with me, then abandons me like

the boys I liked too much in high school. I
watch his white coat flapping behind him as he
leaves.

Another day, another dollar.

A Proper Visit

Michele visits me in the hospital.
I notice her black lace-up Sketchers, insist I try
them on. They feel like heaven on my feet.

I ask her if I can have them,
but she says, "No—they are old and smelly."
Tells me they're her *black stinkies*.
By the time I relinquish them
the visiting hour is over.

I beg the staff to let me out
because Michele drove all this way,
and I want a proper visit.

Chelsea Morning

I have my favorite nurses—Katy and Betty,
and I have my favorite technicians too.

Chelsea is funny; she gets me.
I tell her she's my mother hen, that I follow her
around like a little duckling.

I like to sit with her at lunch while she does paperwork. I tell her I'll be quiet so she can grade her papers. Chelsea takes me into the courtyard outside, a slab of cement with walls all around.

We sit and I relish the sun or the breeze, all those things one takes for granted.

Each morning I look for her, knowing that if she's here it'll be a better day.

Detox

Many patients are admitted here to detox from drugs or alcohol.

My roommate, Marilyn, is in her fifties, sports a red bob, and often forgets to flush the toilet. She sleeps a lot too, even though we're not supposed to nap. She came in not long ago from a night of binge drinking and now it is her time to go home.

Before she leaves, my roommate asks me to sign her AA Bible. The large tome has already been signed in several places.

It takes me awhile to locate a blank spot.

Art Therapy

There are two dayrooms in the unit.
I prefer the smaller one where we can listen to
music.

Mark, who suffers from depression, finds solace
in listening to my John Denver CDs. He sits on
the floor hugging his knees to his chest.

"You seem too young to like the same kind of
music as I do," he says. I invite him to come
sit with us as we draw at the table where I'm
tracing my hands.

Kayla, a young, anxious patient, is coloring a
picture for her sister. Drawing calms her down.

Mark selects a red implement, sketches a rose
with precision. Then suddenly he tosses the
colored pencil nub in the plastic tub with
disgust. "I can't draw," he laments.

Kayla asks if he's mad at us, as he curls into
a fetal position on the floor.
"No," I say. "Not at us."

Taking Three for the Kids

Sometimes my pharmaceutical cocktail is so

strong, especially the one I take at night,
I feel buzzed going to bed.

Nurse Katy always lets me look up the names
of the drugs in her handbook.

One night Nurse Katy isn't working and a nurse
I've never met gives me unfamiliar pills.

I tell him I don't want them, but he says,
"What about your sons? Would you take them
for their sake?"

I tell him it's like he's giving me a shot, but I
think about the boys, and swallow the three
capsules down.

My Other Favorite Technician

Shayne, my other favorite technician, knows
when to suggest to the nurses I need some
lorazepam to calm down.

He always approaches me when I cry. If it's in
the cafeteria he unlocks the bathroom door for
me so I can collect myself.

But he puts it to me straight too. One day in
recreational therapy I get frustrated with the
writing assignment, frustrated with asylum in

general. I crumple my paper and toss it in the trash.

He tells me that's not the kind of behavior that'll get me home. I retrieve the mangled page, finish my work.

Going Postal

In the description of patient rights,
it says we have access to send and receive mail.
I take full advantage of this right by sending
letters to my former professor and writing to the
prison pen-pal I have through a church ministry.

I never hear back from either one of them.

Reinforcements

The cafeteria is decorated for St. Patrick's Day, which is today, and I do feel lucky because tomorrow I get to go home.

This time, though, Dr. Peterson wants reinforcements—extended family to be involved. We make a plan. I'll stay at the lake cottage with Aunt Jane and Uncle Terry for a week, then, over spring break, Rick will bring the boys.

Mom and Bob still have their cottage next to Jane's, so we can all spread out.

Dr. Peterson says people with bipolar can benefit from being by a lake.

Respect

I am losing the respect of my sons.

At dinner the night before I'm to go to the lake, I correct Ayalkbet's manners. He's gobbling down the pizza too fast.

He laughs in my face.

-THIRTEEN-

A Wish

I wish I could tell you that having
reinforcements in place helps, but I am still off
my chain.

Beautiful Day

It's the second day Rick and the boys are at the
lake. The water looks like glass. The sun is out.
I dress quickly and clip my iPod to my jeans.

My family is sleeping in Mom's cottage
because I feel safer from Rick at Aunt Jane's.
He's put me in the hospital too many times,
and I'm not going to let it happen again.

As I walk towards Mom's cabin, I stop to prop a
toy guitar from Aunt Jane's house against a post
to mark my presence.

Inside the cottage, there's a CD player on a table
by the oak cabinet. I put on a compilation, a
tribute of songs about 9/11 from various artists.

Rick emerges, yelling, "Your boys are asleep!"
turns off Springsteen.

When I leave, I take a cowboy hat with me,
place it on the fence between the two properties.

There's a single fishing boat on the lake, and
I'm pretty sure it's a guy named Stan whom I
used to work with at the assisted living home.
He likes to fish. As I'm watching Stan, the song,
"Another One Bites the Dust" plays on my iPod,
and I begin to dance.

Next, I read some Emily Dickinson poems.
One about how "surgeons must be very careful
when they take the knife" catches my eye.
I decide this is about me and Dr. Peterson,
head inside, email it to him.

Then I call Julie, my good friend to whom I
haven't spoken in a decade, leave a voicemail
describing what a beautiful day it is.

The Nap

I spend the remainder of the afternoon

128

walking back and forth between the two cottages. By about 3 p.m. my feet hurt so bad, I am hobbling.

"Mom, lay down," orders Yakob. I lie down on a twin bed on Mom's covered porch, then spring back up.

Yakob tells me to stay, removing my shoes. "When can I get back up?" I ask, giggling. He covers me with a blanket.

The Trade

During the week the lake gets busier. I see that Obama's secret servicemen have arrived.

I also apply to graduate school for environmental education, and send Michele a letter telling her I'll trade her my wedding ring for her black stinkies.

In the evenings, by the seawall, I hold my lighter up, signaling the writer, Tom Robbins, who I'm sure lives across the lake.

Tears

It is the last day at the lake. Rick and I are in the kitchen arguing about the graffiti I've written

with black marker on the back of my silver
Honda Pilot and Mom's antique oak cabinet.
I had written variations of the f-word among
other things. He also demands to know why I've
been throwing lighters in the lake. "Are you
ever going to take that thing off?" he asks.
To spite him, I turn up the offending iPod.

"What about your family?" asks Rick.
Yakob enters the room.
"Yeah, Mom, what about your family? What
about us?"

There are tears in his eyes I'll never forget.

Just Like When I Was a Kid

My sons help me clean the graffiti as we prepare
to leave the lake. Ayalkbet works the hardest to
erase my words.

Although the plan is for me to go back to
Franklin with Rick, I'm scared to get in the car
with him. So I ride with Aunt Jane and Terry
to my parents' primary residence in Carmel.

For about a week I live with Mom and Bob,
get in trouble for taking Mom's car without
permission, just like when I was a kid.

The Hand-off

I don't want to go with Rick when my parents
hand me off at a Fazoli's half-way to Franklin.

They make me take lorazepam for the ride.
They are upset and take one too.

My First Clue

Back home I "sleep" on the couch, taking
pictures of our living room all night, reading my
professor's blog, adding my own comments, and
listening to my iPod.

Rick takes me to the hospital in the morning,
says I just have an appointment. My first clue
that I'm in for more than a check-up is that it's a
Sunday. During the ride, I turn up Sheryl Crow,
scream out the window how "I'm still the king
of me."

I'm alone in the waiting room when Dr.
Peterson sticks his head in the doorway, says,
"You've lost a lot of weight," then disappears.

Upstairs Ann, the weekend nursing supervisor,
is standing at the desk. "I'm not very happy to
see you," I tell her. "That's ok," she says calmly.

A patient who looks like Jim Morrison after a
rough night, walks up to me, stares in my eyes,
and shouts, "Whore!" Before I can respond
Nurse Katy calls me over, tells me she has my
lorazepam.

"I don't need any lorazepam.
He's the one who called me a whore."
"I have an order from your doctor to give you a
shot if you don't take it. You don't want a shot,
do you?"

I tell her I'm in here for listening to my iPod
too much. Then I take the small white pill, sleep
through dinner.

I'm still groggy at night, go to bed, and pray that
someone nice will be working in the morning.

Losing My Religion

I demand spiritual counsel. It's one of our
patient rights. Rick calls the Catholic church we
sometimes attend.

Father Bali, whom I've never met, agrees to
come. He arrives one evening, wearing a brown
robe with a white belt. His eyes exude warmth.

I explain to Father that I feel I'll never get to go

132

home and that I'm not getting along with my husband.

Father reaches into a pocket, gives me a white, round container. On the top is a picture of Mary holding her hands outward with palms open. "For you," he says, with what sounds like an Indian accent.

I twist open the top. Inside is a wooden rosary, the beads stained fuchsia in color.

"Thank you," I say, running my fingers over the beads.
"I speak to your husband. He is good, I think," he says.

Linda, a new patient with white bandages around her wrists, peeks in the room. I invite her to pray with us. Then we gather other patients.

"We're going to church," I tell Molly, a technician who sits at the nurses' station working a crossword puzzle.

During prayer, Father focuses on the healings Jesus performed for the sick.
He offers the Catholics communion, gives the others who aren't Catholic rosaries instead.

When he leaves, I feel a calm I haven't felt in a long while. Then Molly confiscates our rosaries, considers them a form of jewelry. We aren't allowed to have jewelry.

I gaze at my empty, white container with Mary's picture on it.

Pretty Stones

I miss my sons. When I write to Ayalkbet, who loves rocks, I tape some pebbles from the courtyard to the letter.

The pretty stones are all I have to offer.

Commune

I like to give things away.

Chris, a young man who speaks with a slight lisp, gets my John Lennon t-shirt, and quiet Sharon, who wears long coppery wigs, can have a pair of my shoes.

One evening, when the night nurse catches on, she holds group, says it needs to stop, that "we're not running a commune around here."

The next day is a bad one. I want to go home.

When I see the same yuppie nurse from group the night before, I tell her in a wavering voice that I don't appreciate her comment about the commune. She all but rolls her eyes at me, which really pisses me off.

P.S. Panty Snatcher

I'm doing laps around the nurses' station when a technician approaches me, holding up a plastic baggie for my view. Inside is my pair of underwear, the green ones with the gold stripes. They're one of my Christmas panties. She asks me to identify them, and I do.

They were found in Chris's room. This makes me feel violated and curious as to how he got them, because we're not allowed in our rooms during the day.

P.S. I want my John Lennon t-shirt back.

Insurance

Angie weighs about 95 pounds, wears a fleece farm coat on most days. She speaks with her head down, shaking it from side to side, creating the effect she isn't talking to me but to an imaginary friend. She is prone to laughing fits and bouts of sadness or irritability. Her moods sometimes coincide with my own.

One day Angie tells me she was smoking four
packs a day before coming here.

"Did they give you the patch?" I ask.
"They said something about how
insurance wouldn't pay," she laments.

I plead her case for the patch to all the doctors,
because I'm lucky to have insurance and she
doesn't, and because I've been in here so long
I'm sort of acting like a barn boss.

I think about what Dr. Peterson once said—
about how I'm better off than most of the
patients here.

A Joke

I've been in this place for so long I see a
building on the property go up from floor to
frame.

I joke with Chelsea that I'm paying for the
construction, only when I really think about it,
it isn't very funny.

Recovery

When I do get to go home, Rick picks me up.
I've been through this so many times, I'm
relieved, but not happy.

My recovery is slow, not only mentally, but
physically as well. I get a headache about every
twelve hours, I assume from going off the patch.
My frontal lobe tingles at times. I discover I can
make it stop by listening to my iPod.

When I get on the computer, it's like plodding
through quicksand. Bright lights bother me.
I'm tired because you don't have to do a lot in
the hospital. It's like I have atrophied.

Resilient

It's awkward at first around the boys, who look
to Rick now for their needs. But children are
resilient, with a capacity to forgive and forget
that is deeper than in most adults.

Return to Sender

In fact, when I go through my email sent box,
cringing at what I'd written, which included a
poem about my menstrual cycle I had sent to
our sons' soccer coach, I attempt to apologize to

a couple of people, only to discover they have blocked me. It feels like a swift kick to the gut.

-FOURTEEN-

He Doesn't Know Me

I notice later in my release paperwork that I have four diagnoses: bipolar I, anxiety, mixed p.d., and marital problems.

I don't know what a mixed p.d. is but later discover it means I have a mixed personality disorder. This bothers me to no end because it's ambiguous, and I take it personally—

But then I remember what one of the technicians told us in group, about how a diagnosis can change, and once you have been labeled something, it doesn't mean you'll always be that. I decide he's right. The person my doctor knows from the hospital is not the person I am. He doesn't know the funny me, the creative me, or the compassionate me.

He only knows the me who was very sick.

Fifty Days

If I do the math, my total hospitalizations over this past winter and spring add up to around fifty days. I do not know why it took so long for my symptoms to subside.

I do know that during those fifty days, I missed my sons' spring soccer season and seeing Ayalkbet play the real Barack Obama in the presidential school play, not the one who was a figment of my imagination.

And I tested the mettle of my marriage almost more than it could bear.

What Goes Up, Must Come Down

Often bipolar disorder is like the law of gravity: what goes up, must come down.

I spend most of the summer following my hospitalizations in a terrible haze, which had actually started to sink in during the last few days of my asylum.

As despair thickens, I pass the slow tick of time on the back deck hunched over at the table,

feeling old. I call my friends but have nothing
to say and yet feel an odd sort of comfort in the
silence that hangs between us, just knowing they
are on the other end of the phone.

I try to help around the house, but filling a pot
with water for spaghetti requires Herculean
effort, and all I want to do is go back outside,
to sit.

What's Bugging Me

My outpatient doctor is retiring, and since
I've been recently hospitalized, I have trouble
finding a doctor outside Peterson who will work
with me.

And when I do, he prescribes something that
makes my urine dark and my legs feel like there
are bugs crawling inside the skin.

Baby Steps

The tinkering of meds is a slow process.
While I'm on the healing journey, I find myself
getting a few things done each day.

But this is a tedious road, and it's hard
being an adult who can only take baby steps.

Discoveries

Memories of my madness turn up at random
times. While dusting, I find a copy of the book
I thought my professor had penned about me
hidden in the back of a bookshelf.

When I check the mail, I notice a sticky goo
crawling with ants. I had poured green tea inside
the mailbox to christen it in anticipation of a
letter of acceptance from a book publisher.

More clues turn up in the bushes. My box
of 1966 US mint coins given to me by my
grandfather are wedged in the juniper bush
against our house. I vaguely recall placing them
there as a gift for a friend.

Each time I make a discovery, it feels like I've
defused a land mine.

Poison in My Pen

I'm writing about the hospital and how my
doctor walked in on me in the bathroom once,
and one of the staff told me to quit using the
hospital as a revolving door (like I enjoyed
being there).

When I share it with my friend, Jim, who is also

a mentor for my writing, he says it's important for me to keep writing about it.

But we both know it's nowhere near publishable. There's too much anger in it, and it lacks the perspective that time gives to any situation.

But poison in my pen or not,
it still feels good to get it out.

Reflections from the Back Porch

I do not know the exact moment when I turned the corner into madness. Perhaps it was when I heard a larger-than-life bird song, or saw amplified colors.

When it became clear Rick could not keep me safe at home, I was hospitalized. There, I found a new sanctuary at a round table in the corner of one of the dayrooms. From my perch, I could look out the window and imagine going home. I colored, wrote letters, and listened to music. But it wasn't the same as our covered deck back home. It lacked privacy. It lacked my kids. I couldn't hear birdsong or the wind through the trees.

But I still have hope.

Now Rick and I sit out here together in the evenings. We especially like it when it is breezy and cool. I have strung lights from the ceiling that cast a comforting glow. I like to think the cherub atop a book knick-knack watches over us. In the yard, our birdhouses sway back and forth if there is a breeze. The trees in the wind seem to whisper, hush, hush.

I do not mention the imprisonment or hospitalization and neither does he. Instead, we talk about our sons, the dogs, his job, my writing. We study the birds. We wait for butterflies.

I hardly ever notice the airplanes.

Back to the Basics

I've been going to the YMCA, and I decide to take my exercise up a notch by enrolling in a boot camp class. I sign Rick up as well.

We have to do planks, run suicide sprints, and race others in the class through obstacle courses. Even though we come in last, I am proud of us just for finishing.

Getting physically active was something we enjoyed when we first started dating. Sometimes in the wake of challenging times, getting back to the basics is a way to rebuild what was lost.

Once More to the Lake

Only time heals the rifts madness creates—
rifts in the self and with others.

We head to the lake for a visit. I don't know
if it's true that all people with bipolar benefit
from being near lakes, but I know that I do. I
note with a fleeting feeling of nostalgia, the lake
looks smaller than it did when I was little.

With me is a new iPod which holds more songs,
but I bring my old one, too. On walks, I listen
to it, searching for clues of what happened last
time we were here, and wonder if the music
enhanced my psychosis.

There are no secret servicemen in sight. I do not
try to signal Tom Robbins. Instead, I watch the
kids fish and ski, observe the floating swans.
I see the sun go down over the water and am
grateful for another day of sanity.

Question

You may wonder if I would rather not have
bipolar disorder.

The trouble is I've had it so long
I don't know any other way.

Stage Mom

Ayalkbet will be home from school soon, and
my heart sinks as I think about telling him the
news. Last night, we had attended an audition
for what we thought was a chance for him to
be on the Miley Cyrus show, and tonight is
supposed to be the final audition. Only today I
did some digging to discover the whole thing is
a scam to sell expensive acting lessons. In our
minds, we had already moved to California and
settled in a mansion.

When he comes home from school, I offer him
cheese and crackers and we go outside so he can
play some basketball. I sit at the little café table
by our driveway and watch as he makes shot
after shot from various distances to the goal.
The only time I can ever come close to doing
this is when I'm manic.

A striker on his travel soccer team, he's an
awesome athlete. But I've always tried to
encourage dabbling in his artistic side.

"You want to play pig, Mom?" he asks.
"Yeah, I'll play," I say.

After he beats me, we go inside for a cold drink.
"You're a great athlete," I say.
"Thanks." He grins.

As we have our water, I think of how I'm going to tell him about the audition. But when I open my mouth, the words, "Do you want to play some more pig?" come out. At the point in the game where I get an "i," I explain that he did well in the audition, but that the company was really just trying to sell acting lessons.

"That's okay," he says, making his next shot. "I'm going to be a basketball pro."

He grins and tosses me the ball.

Maybe if my son can go with the flow when disappointments come, so should I.

To Do

I look to Rusty as a role model. The vet agrees, recently telling my husband that the older rat terriers get, the smarter they seem to be.

One thing I vow to change about my current lifestyle is my to-do list. After filling a page of my notebook as is typical, I have bogged it down with more tasks than I can possibly manage in a day. I combine my current aspirations with what I didn't get done the day before, often making it a two-page list. So it is that each morning I set myself up for failure.

In the meantime, on a typical morning, Rusty is curled in a ball, snuggled against the green, lumpy afghan on our bed. I wake Rusty gently with a few rubs on his head. He slowly stretches, then rolls on his back for tummy rubs. After his massage, I pick him up and carry our little dog outside.

I set him on the deck, and he walks around for a minute before easing down the steps into our yard. Once he finds a good spot to do his business, Rusty does a few laps around the yard for exercise.

Our rat terrier is sitting by the fence, his head pointed high, facing the sun, when I set his dish of food down for him. As Rusty eats, he doesn't scarf it down like Dude and Bear. Nor does he hoard his food like Maggie.

Sleep when you want. Exercise. Take only what you need, leave the rest. Enjoy sunshine on your face. These are some of the rituals that Rusty lives by.

Rusty loves listening to Bob Seger and light rock in general. I keep a radio on the back porch, and he crawls into his pink bed next to it, ears perked toward the music, head cocked.

Rusty likes to frolic. He'll often go up to Dude and get in play stance with his rump in the air, belly down and front paws bouncing against the floor. Dude ignores him, but Rusty doesn't seem to be offended.

In the evenings, when it gets cooler, we place Rusty on his red blanket on the couch. For reasons we can't explain, Rusty enjoys licking the couch, often leaving a wet spot the size of a grapefruit. Perhaps this is how he meditates.

Take naps. Listen to good music. Make time to play. Meditate. These are the things that Rusty could cross off his list if he had one.

I close my notebook on my to-do list, breathe through my nose, out my mouth, and into my belly.

Aripiprazole

The generic name for Abilify is aripiprazole. The real potential side effects according to the package insert include neuroleptic malignant syndrome—a rare and serious condition that can lead to death, high blood sugar, increase in weight, difficulty swallowing, decreased blood pressure, low white blood cell count, seizures, and tardive dyskinesia—a sometimes permanent condition wherein you cannot control movement of the face or other body parts. This can also occur when you stop taking Abilify.

And that's the bitch of some of these psychotropic meds. You take them, but you pray they don't kill you.

The Art of Self-care

I'm still learning the art of consistent self-care. When I get out of balance by working too much, or something happens like a family emergency, my writing, exercise, and attempts at eating nutritious foods fall by the wayside.

I feel like I've hopped on a gerbil wheel.

It gets to a point where I have to reprioritize and start over. I'll schedule an appointment with my life coach, set the timer for fifteen minutes of writing, walk around the block, or eat apple slices with peanut butter.

The Party

I'm having a party, and I'm not sure why.
Maybe it's because I want to feel like I'm really
at home again in my surroundings.

People gather at our house—friends, neighbors,
even our realtor and her husband, and a couple
of patients from the hospital.

There's Angela and Sean who were both there
with me toward the end. They ended up moving
in together.

Sean's an ex-marine. He drinks beer by the
window while Angela and I talk in the garage.

When we come back in, our realtor wants to
know how Angela and I met.

Where to begin?

Home

On the way to our sons' travel soccer game,
we're listening to Elton John.
"And it's good old country comfort in my
bones." I sing along. Yakob and Ayalkbet chime
in. "It's the sweetest sound my ears have ever
known."

Rich colors of fall foliage blanket the trees
along the hilly countryside as we zoom along.

Something about fall drives makes me long for
Indiana, but I know that in this moment, with
my family, I am home.

Graduation

In November 2010, I finish a brief-residency
MFA program at Spalding University in
Louisville, Kentucky. I enrolled in this program
before we moved to Wilmington, and this act of
completion is remarkable because it signifies for
me, that despite the turbulence that sometimes
characterizes my life, long-term goals can be
met.

Workshops during residencies, guided by
gentle sages, were sacred spaces where I shared
writing about my disease with a sort of grace.

Gathered at the celebration are some of the
most important people in my life—both sets of
parents, aunts and uncles, siblings, and friends.
And, especially, Rick and the boys. I can tell our
sons are impressed by the whole shebang.

At Spalding, all graduating students must read
some of their work aloud. As I look out at a sea

of my supporters, I read a fitting story about
Thanksgiving and being grateful for all of the
important things in life—like water and shelter,
full bellies and laughter,
health and reinforcements.

Life itself.

EPILOGUE

It's been six years since my series of four hospitalizations. I still go to my aunt's lake cottage taking time to write and reflect when I can. There are a few pieces of jewelry I'd flung into the woods behind her house while manic, which I'd like to find. I imagine the patina of the metal has tarnished with time. Or maybe a young woman, facing her own struggles, found a necklace, and it brightened her day.

As a scared adolescent locked on a psychiatric ward, I saw ominous ravens in the sky. Later, as an adult, I witnessed doppelgangers and angels in the grocery store. It turns out they weren't real, but angels bless me every day. My husband, Rick, is very patient. My stepdaughters and their families, our sons and brave daughter from Haiti, who now completes our family, add rich layers to my life. Thank God for our pets, too. I have so much to be grateful for, including being balanced.

I'm thinking about any advice I can give to others with bipolar disorder. The sweetness of time has been my saving grace. It's important to hold on to the fact that even while in the pit of despair, things will change. You will not be manic or depressed forever. Make good use of the times between both extremes of mood, but don't put pressure on yourself.

I've learned that mental illness makes some people uncomfortable, and I've lost friends through this. If this happens to you, let them go. Cherish what remains. My friends are the best you could hope for.

Having a sense of humor helps. I think it's funny that my aunt kept hearing a beeping sound in the woods long after my episode. She followed the noise to discover a watch of mine.

Pharmacology and therapy play a huge role in successful treatment of the disease. If your therapist falls asleep on you, find a new one. Selecting a psychiatrist is like finding the perfect pair of jeans. It has to be a good fit. Medications and dosages may need to be tinkered with for a while before relief comes. Don't tinker with them on your own like I did.
Writing is also a form of medicine.

Although it can be a challenge to keep the habit, exercise can be invaluable in helping regulate moods. We are designed to create our own feel-good chemicals. Listening to familiar, well-liked music can release dopamine. I like dancing in my kitchen. Additionally, I try to eat well and get a good night's sleep. This advice is nothing new, and yet so important. And lastly, approaching life with a spirit of gratitude helps. If something good happens, take note of it.

When you are feeling on an even-keel, you can "harness it for good" as one of my doctors once advised me, whatever that means to you.
For me it was writing this book.

And yet bipolar disorder is a chronic condition. There will come a time when optimism gives way to despair, or I see doppelgangers again. All I can do is my best. That's all any of us can do.

ABOUT THE AUTHOR

Colleen Wells lives in Bloomington, Indiana, with her husband and three children. Her work has appeared in *Adoptive Families Magazine*, *Chicken Soup for the Adoptive Soul*, *NUVO*, *ORION*, *Georgetown Review*, and *Potomac Review* among other publications. In 2002 she was the recipient of a first place award from the Indiana Chapter of The Society of Professional Journalists for her feature "Road Kill—Casualties of the Car Culture" which appeared in *NUVO*. She holds a BA in English from Indiana University, an MA in English from Butler University, and an MFA in Creative Writing from Spalding University. She has worked in several schools and colleges in various roles including as an adjunct faculty member, tutor, and teaching assistant.

RESOURCES

According to the National Institute of Mental Health and NAMI (National Alliance on Mental Illness), 2.6 percent of American adults have bipolar disorder. I'm one of them. That statistic means I'm one of 6.1 million in the United States alone. And yet as far as statistics go, I consider myself lucky as there's a high percentage of people with mental illness who also experience homelessness, incarceration, or a lack of mental health services.

The internet has a wealth of information about bipolar disorder. Here are just a handful of websites where you can read more.

American Foundation for Suicide Prevention
www.afsp.org

Bipolar Child Support
www.bipolarchildsupport.com

BP Hope: Hope and Harmony for People with Bipolar
www.bphope.com

Depression and Bipolar Support Alliance
www.dbsalliance.org

Esperanza: Hope to Cope with Anxiety and Depression
www.hopetocope.com

International Bipolar Foundation
www.ibpf.org

International Society for Bipolar Disorders
www.isbd.org

National Alliance on Mental Illness
www.nami.org

The Balanced Mind
www.thebalancedmind.org

National Institute of Mental Health
www.nimh.nih.gov/health/topics/bipolar-disorder/index.shtml

Find wholesale prices at the

wordpoolpress.com

Other titles from Wordpool Press:

Seventh of Eleven
by Dorothy Sabean

The Omega Principle
by Bill De Herder

 Find Wordpool Press on Facebook!